Total Hip Replacement

Kalliopi Lampropoulou-Adamidou
George Hartofilakidis

Total Hip Replacement

Case Series from a Leading Registry

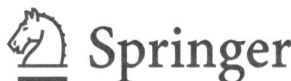 Springer

Kalliopi Lampropoulou-Adamidou
Laboratory for the Research of
Musculoskeletal System
"Th. Garofalidis", Medical School
National and Kapodistrian University
of Athens
KAT General Hospital of Athens
Athens
Greece

George Hartofilakidis
Laboratory for the Research of
Musculoskeletal System
"Th. Garofalidis", Medical School
National and Kapodistrian University
of Athens
KAT General Hospital of Athens
Athens
Greece

ISBN 978-3-319-53359-9   ISBN 978-3-319-53360-5   (eBook)
DOI 10.1007/978-3-319-53360-5

Library of Congress Control Number: 2017941255

Printed on acid-free paper

This Springer imprint is published by Springer Nature
The registered company is Springer International Publishing AG
The registered company address is: Gewerbestrasse 11, 6330 Cham, Switzerland

Total hip replacement demands respect from both the orthopaedic surgeon and the patient.

George Hartofilakidis

Foreword

The book by Dr. Kalliopi Lampropoulou-Adamidou and Professor George Hartofilakidis entitled *Total Hip Replacement: Case Series from a Leading Registry* is a timely, comprehensive and practical contribution to the orthopaedic literature. Any practicing orthopaedic surgeon can unequivocally state that despite the long history of total hip replacement, we still are witnessing marked changes in its indications and techniques. For this reason, there is a clear need to critically analyze the available information to help surgeons make sound treatment decisions.

Total hip replacement has been one of the most widely used and successful innovations in modern orthopaedic reconstructive surgery, and with the current aging population, orthopaedic surgeons of the next decades will be asked to perform a growing number of primary procedures and revision surgeries. This book greatly facilitates a practical learning experience by teaching in a case-based manner, providing the reader with real cases to improve their comprehension of the intricacies of total hip replacement surgery.

While many books have been published on total hip replacement, this book represents one of the only substantial series of educational cases. Cases, such as the one collected in this volume, provide the surgeon with detailed information and help to underscore the tips and pearls related to total hip replacement. The specific case studies in this volume are derived from an invaluable registry of clinical cases performed by Professor George Hartofilakidis, a renowned expert in hip replacement. Case studies from a comprehensive registry, such as this, provide valuable teaching material, demonstrating both classical and unusual presentation, which may confront the surgeon.

Professor Hartofilakidis and Dr. Lampropoulou-Adamidou have done a superb job of selecting educational cases covering state-of-the-art knowledge in total hip replacement. This book provides comprehensive evidence-based information on total hip replacement and I am confident that it will be very useful for experienced orthopaedic surgeons, residents and fellows to comprehend and apply total hip replacement techniques for the effective management of their patients.

Orthopaedic Research & Education Center   Panayotis N. Soucacos, MD, FACS
Attikon University Hospital
National & Kapodistrian University of Athens
School of Medicine
Athens, Greece

.

Preface

The Orthopaedic Department of University of Athens was one of the first centres in Greece where total hip replacement (THR) was introduced into clinical practice. The majority of complicated cases and neglected or maltreated cases of congenital hip disease (CHD) in infancy were referred to that centre for treatment. Our THR Registry was established in the early 1970s. It includes approximately 1000 THRs, performed by one surgeon (GH) from 1973 to 1994 and followed continuously.

The core idea of this book is to provide, through figures ("a picture is worth more than a thousand words"), orthopaedic surgeons, interested in hip reconstruction surgery, with data from a leading registry, including unique, homogenous information from long-term followed patients.

Many cases are presented with series of preoperative radiographs indicating the natural history of the underlying pathology. In certain cases of CHD, previous radiographs since early childhood are available.

The book presents various cases as a presentation album rather than a conventional textbook. Each case is presented with a short introduction, followed by selected radiographs from different time periods, providing key messages and lessons learned. To our knowledge there is no other book in the field of orthopaedics structured this way.

Cases of low-friction arthroplasty (LFA) with 35–42 years' survival are presented in Chap. 1, indicating the unique potential of this procedure. It is to be noted that even cases with some technical imperfections had unexpectedly long survival. This is an indication that unpredictable parameters may influence the longevity of a THR. Chapter 2 includes cases of THR in patients with CHD treated in infancy in other institutions with late closed reduction and prolonged immobilisation in plaster. Chapter 3 includes cases of THR in patients with CHD who had been previously treated with an osteotomy.

High dislocation is the most severe type of CHD. Special considerations concerning the two subtypes, C1 and C2, of high dislocation are presented in Chap. 4. In Chaps. 5, 6 and 7, selected cases of THR in patients with idiopathic osteoarthritis, inflammatory arthritis and osteonecrosis of the femoral head are illustrated.

Chapter 8 includes cases that remind that THR may involve unexpected disappointment. Therefore, it is imperative to be decided when it is absolutely necessary. Chapter 9 includes cases with special interest. Key messages and lessons learned from this long experience with THR are presented in the final chapter.

The minimum radiographic follow-up of the presented primary THRs of all cases included in the book is 20 years. We would like to thank the members of our team Professor George A. Babis and Assistant Professor John Vlamis for their valuable contribution by performing the majority of the revision operations included in the presented cases.

Athens, Greece   Kalliopi Lampropoulou-Adamidou
Athens, Greece   George Hartofilakidis

Contents

1 Long-Term Survival (35–42 Years)   1

2 Late Closed Reduction in Patients with Congenital
   Hip Disease 19

3 Previous Osteotomies in Patients with Congenital
   Hip Disease 31

4 High Dislocation: C1 and C2 Subtypes 41

5 Idiopathic Osteoarthritis 63

6 Inflammatory Arthritis 71

7 Avascular Necrosis of the Femoral Head 83

8 Complicated Cases 93

9 Miscellaneous 115

Appendix: Key Messages and Lessons Learned 145

The pioneer of total hip replacement (THR), John Charnley, introducing his new method, wrote 55 years ago: "Neither surgeons nor engineers will ever make an artificial hip joint which will last 30 years". His prediction was not confirmed. This revolutionary method, low-friction arthroplasty (LFA), has already survived more than 40 years, while newer methods of THR promise even better results, although there is not yet a universal agreement as to which method of fixation of a THR, cemented, uncemented or hybrid, has the longest survival prospects.

THR is considered as the operation of the century; however, we should not forget that it may involve unexpected disappointment. Therefore, it is of great importance to be decided when there is an absolute indication for THR, based on patients' symptoms, psychological impact, clinical findings and the potential of development of the disorder in each case. Orthopaedic surgeons should protect this operation from the overuse. The patients should be informed for the severity of the procedure, the possible complications and the necessary postoperative adaptations of their daily life.

Although some THRs present several risk factors of a non-favourable outcome, related to the patient or the surgical technique, they may survive more than 35 years. This is an indication that we cannot safely predict the outcome of a THR with the known data. Constant follow-up remains the most reliable way to detect early signs of failure and application of early intervention, before extensive bone damage makes revision difficult, necessitating more complicated surgical techniques.

© Springer International Publishing AG 2017
K. Lampropoulou-Adamidou, G. Hartofilakidis, *Total Hip Replacement*,
DOI 10.1007/978-3-319-53360-5_1

1.1   Case 1

This female patient was born in 1922 with congenital hip disease (CHD) bilaterally. She had no treatment in infancy. She was slightly limping since early infancy, and she started having pain around the age of 25 years. She had a gradual deterioration since that time. We first examined her when she was 52 years old. She had advanced secondary osteoarthritis (OA) in both hips due to low dislocation. She was limping heavily and had severe pain in both hips. LFA was performed in 1974 and 1975 in the left and right hip, respectively. The patient, at the age of 94 years, has an ordinary life with a level of activity compatible to her age, a slight limp and painless hips (Figs. 1.1–1.4).

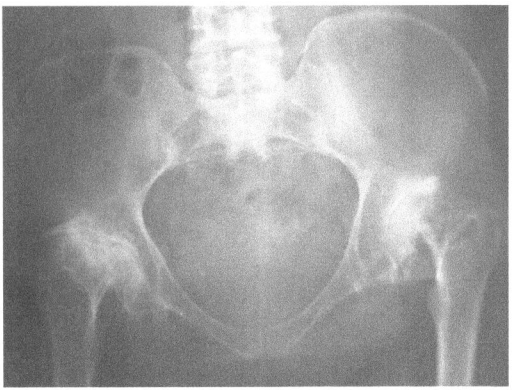

Fig. 1.1 Preoperative radiograph, when the patient was 52 years old

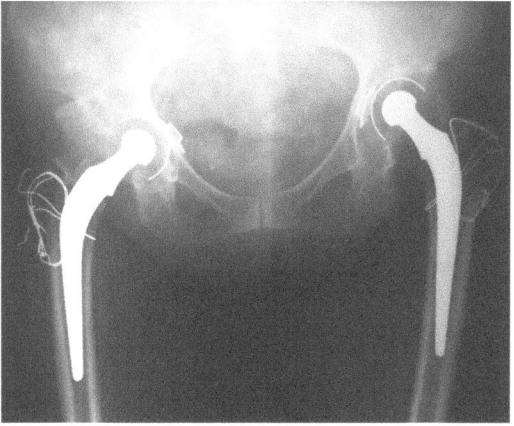

Fig. 1.3 Twenty-five years postoperatively. The patient remained fully active

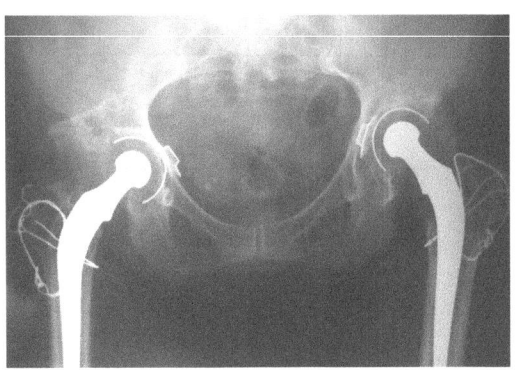

Fig. 1.2 Ten years postoperatively. The cement mantle is not visible because radiopaque barium was not in use at that time

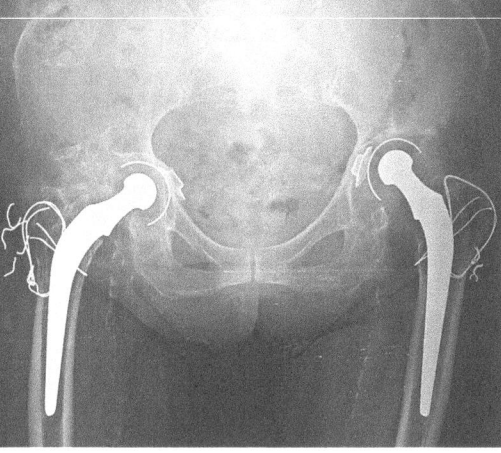

Fig 1.4 The latest follow-up radiograph taken 42 and 41 years after primary THRs of the left and right hip, respectively, when the patient was 94 years old

1.2   Case 2

This female patient was born in 1922. She started complaining of pain in the right hip around the age of 50 years. She had rapid worsening and LFA was performed 3 years later, in 1975. Eight years later, in 1983, she started having pain in the left hip, because of the development of medial eccentric idiopathic OA. LFA of the left hip was performed in 1989, when the patient was 67 years old. Last follow-up evaluation was performed 40 and 26 years after LFA of the right and left hip, respectively, when the patient was 93 years old having a satisfactory level of activity and painless hips (Figs. 1.5–1.8).

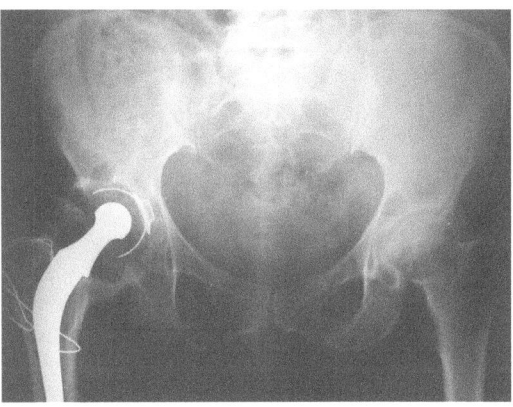

Fig. 1.5 Radiograph taken in 1976, 1 year after LFA of the right hip (the preoperative radiograph was missing). The left hip, with an early stage eccentric idiopathic OA of the medial subtype, was painless

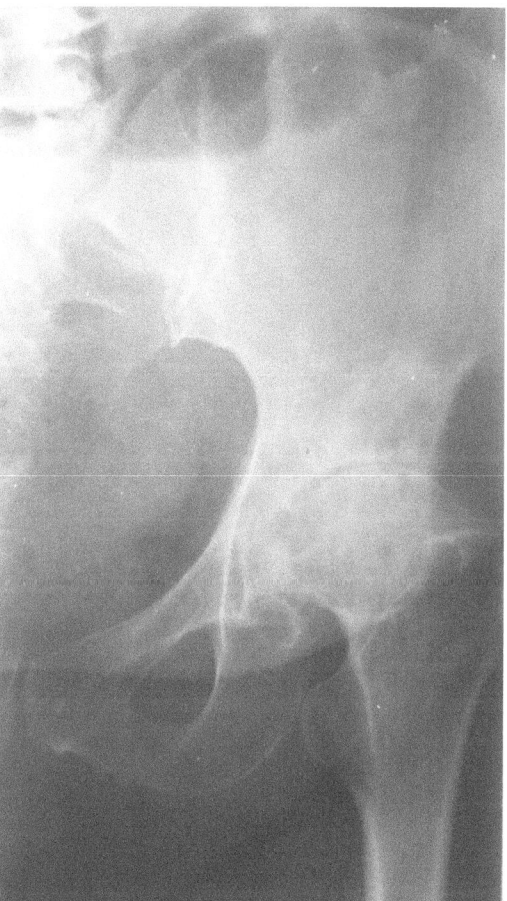

Fig. 1.6 Radiograph taken 9 years later, in 1985. The patient had slight pain in the left hip

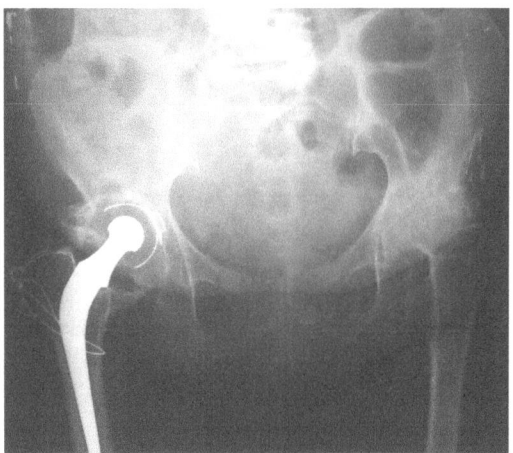

Fig. 1.7 In 1989, 14 years after LFA of the right hip. The left hip presented advanced OA and LFA was followed

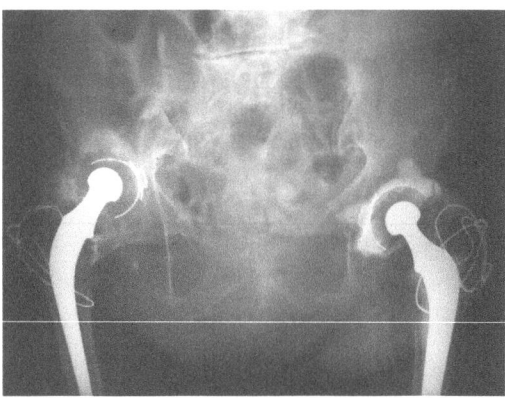

Fig. 1.8 The latest follow-up radiograph 40 and 26 years after primary LFAs of the right and left hip, respectively. Despite radiographic deterioration, it was decided to not advise further surgery, taking patient's advanced age and clinical findings into consideration

1.3   Case 3

This female patient was born in 1932. Around the age of 40 years, she began to have pain in both hips. We examined her when she was 45 years old. Eccentric idiopathic OA of both hips was diagnosed. In 1980, LFA was performed in the left and the right hip within 6 months, when the patient was 48 years old. The last follow-up radiograph was taken 36 years postoperatively. The patient, 84 years old at that time, had both hips asymptomatic and a good activity level (Figs. 1.9–1.12).

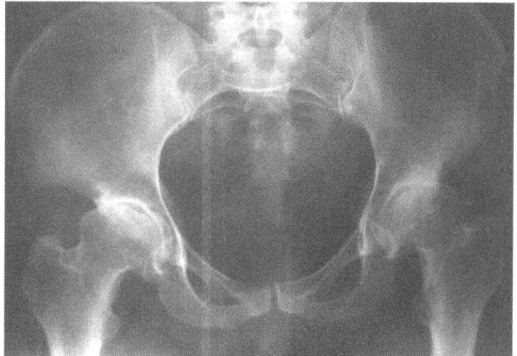

Fig. 1.9 Radiograph when the patient was 45 years old

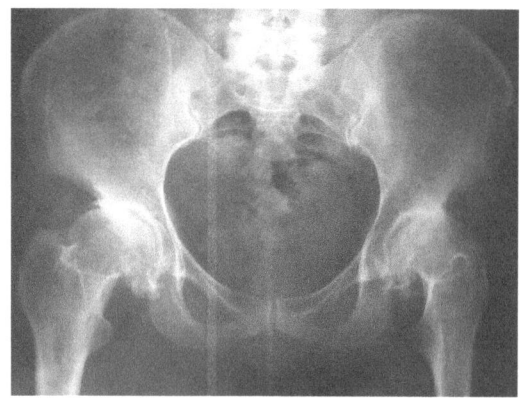

Fig. 1.10 Radiograph 3 years later. Note the rapid progression of degenerative changes

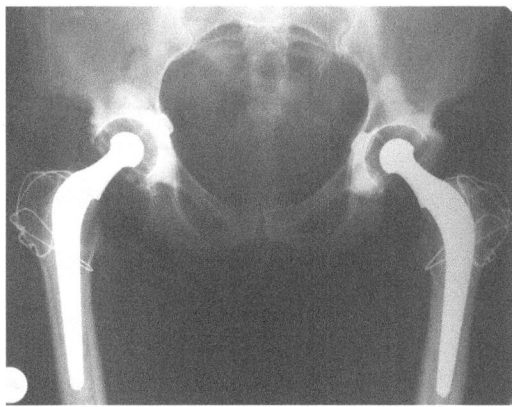

Fig. 1.11 Five years after LFA of both hips performed in 1980

1.4   Case 4

This female patient was born in 1933. At the age of 3 years, she was treated by her physician with closed reduction and prolonged plaster immobilisation for bilateral CHD. She was limping since then, and around the age of 30 years, she started complaining of hip pain. We examined her in 1978, when she was 45 years old. She had bilateral dysplastic hips with severe epiphyseal deformities, especially in the right hip. Pain was also more severe in the right hip and she was limping heavily. At the same year, LFA was performed in the right hip and 10 years later in the left. At the last evaluation, when the patient was 82 years old, 37 and 27 years following LFAs of the right and left hip, respectively, she had no pain or limp, retaining satisfactory activity level. Low back pain was her main complaint (Figs. 1.13–1.20).

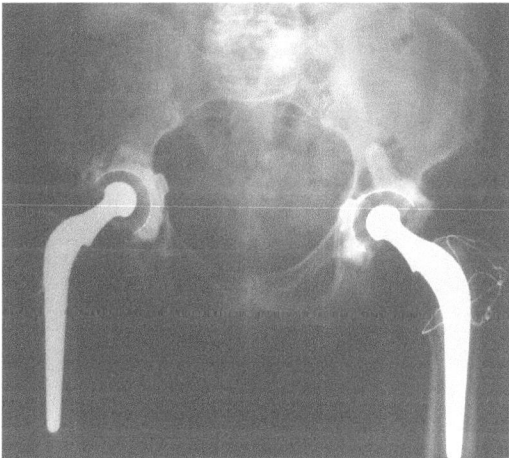

Fig. 1.12 The latest follow-up radiograph taken 36 years after primary LFA

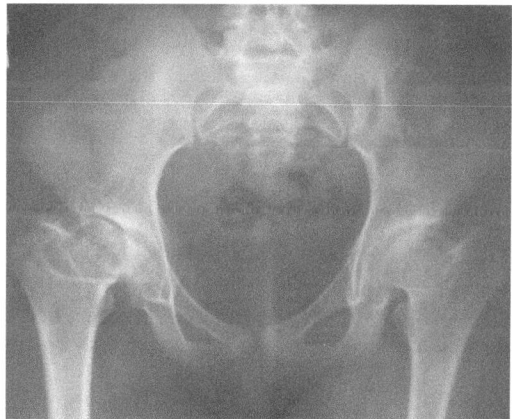

Fig. 1.13 The first available radiograph, when the patient was 15 years old. She was limping, but she had no hip pain

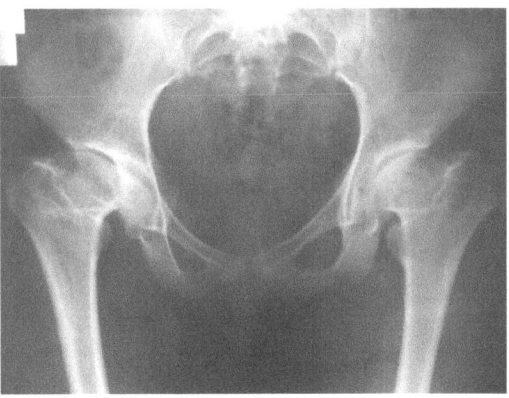

Fig. 1.14 Radiograph, when she was 22 years old and started to have slight pain in the right hip

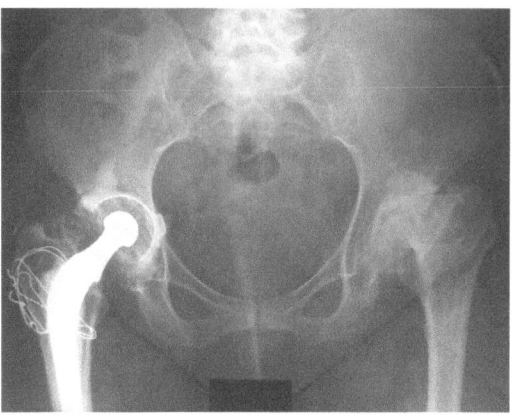

Fig 1.17 Radiograph taken in 1988, 10 years after LFA of the right hip. LFA of the left hip was followed

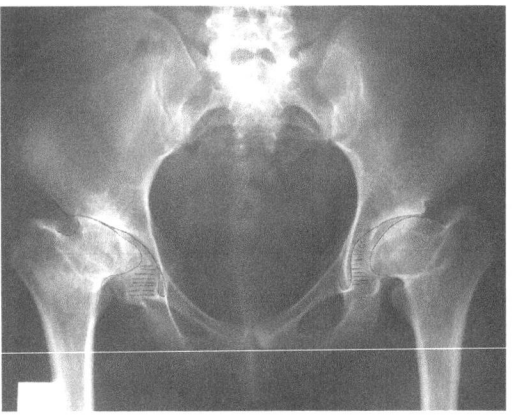

Fig. 1.15 Right hip pain had increased when she was 35 years old

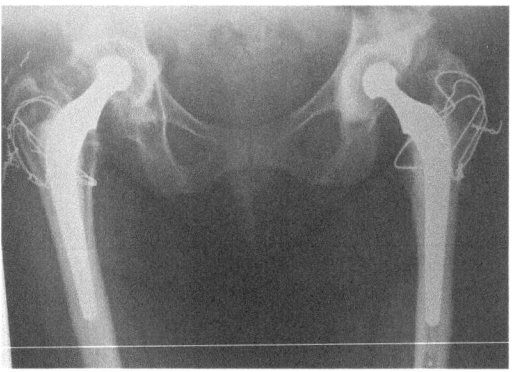

Fig. 1.18 Radiograph taken 25 years after LFA of the right hip and 15 years of the left

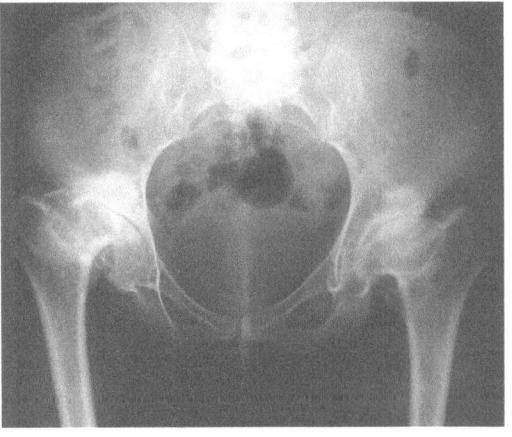

Fig. 1.16 Radiograph taken in 1978 when she was 45 years old and we first examined her. LFA of the right hip was followed

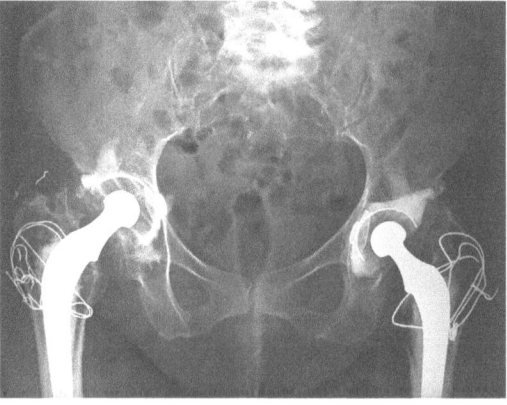

Fig 1.19 The latest follow-up radiograph taken 37 and 27 years after primary replacement of the right and left hip, respectively

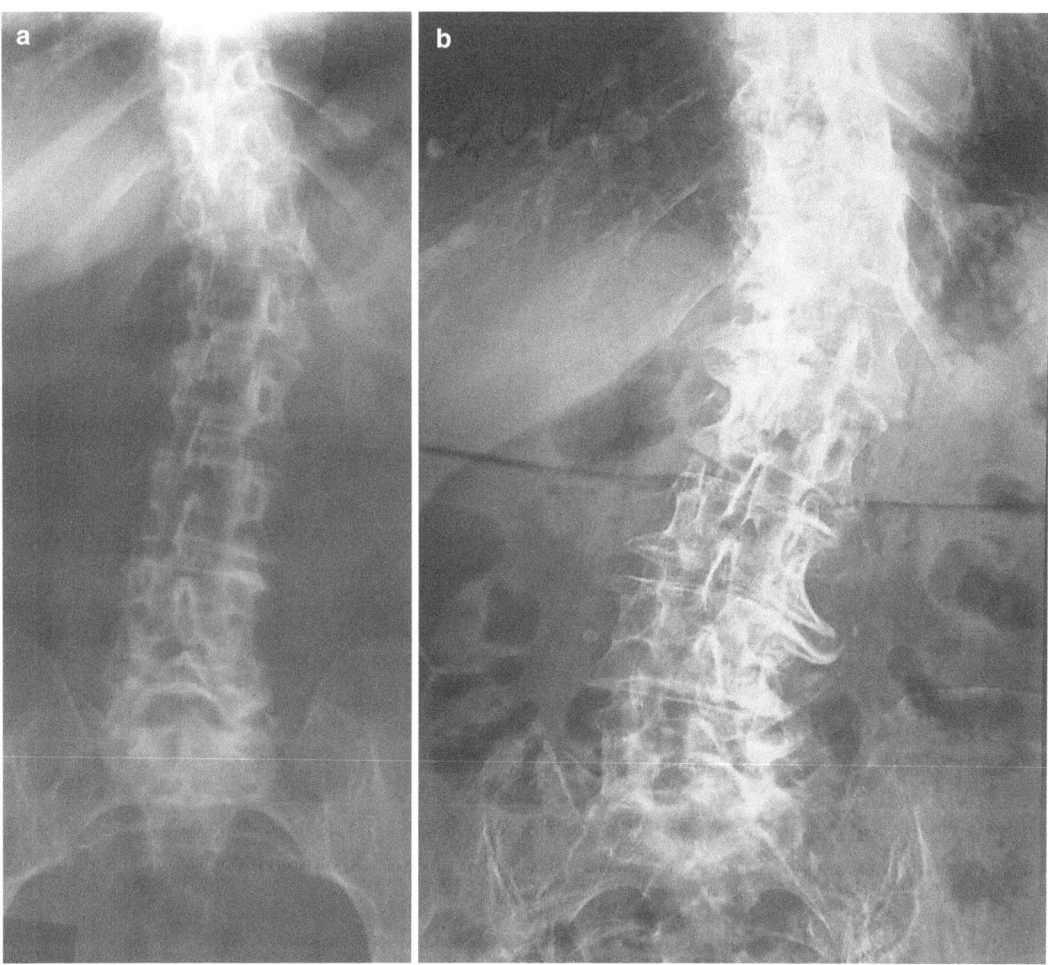

Fig. 1.20 Radiographs of the lumbar spine, when the patient was (**a**) 58 and (**b**) 81 years old. Recent years, severe low back pain was her main complaint

1.5   Case 5

This male patient was born in 1950. He was diagnosed with ankylosing spondylitis at the age of
18 years. Both hips were replaced because of
severe pain and functional disability, in 1976,
when he was 26 years old. For many years, he
was working free of hip pain and was fully active.
Thirty-two years postoperatively, right stem
fractured and a revision of both components was
followed. At the last follow-up examination,
36 years after primary replacement of the left hip
and 5 years after revision of the right when the
patient was 63 years old, he remained asymptomatic and had normal activities (Figs. 1.21–1.25).

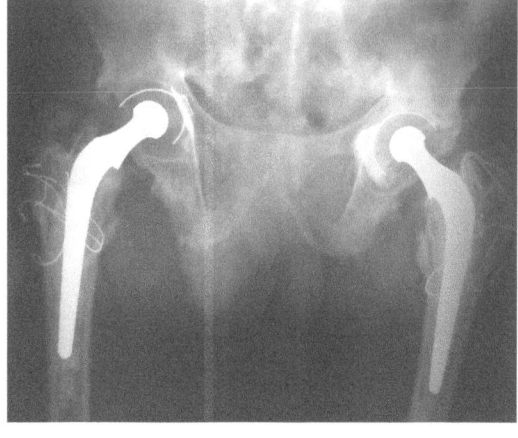

Fig. 1.23 Eighteen years postoperatively

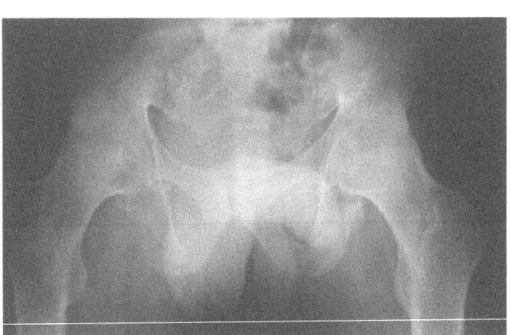

Fig. 1.21 Preoperative radiograph

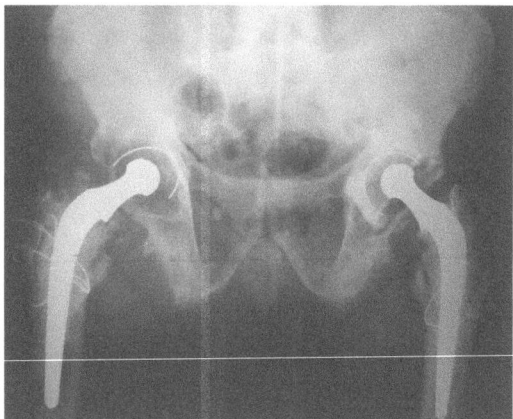

Fig. 1.24 Thirty-two years postoperatively, when the
right stem was fractured

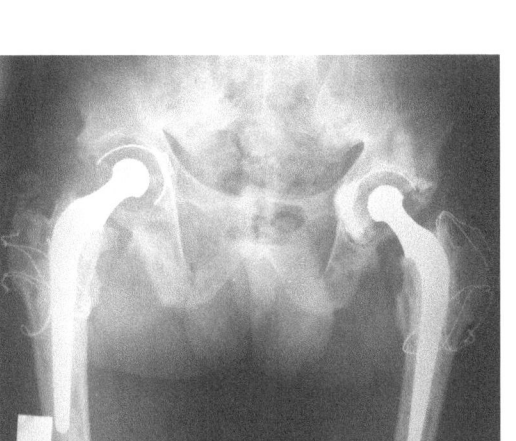

Fig. 1.22 Eight years after LFAs

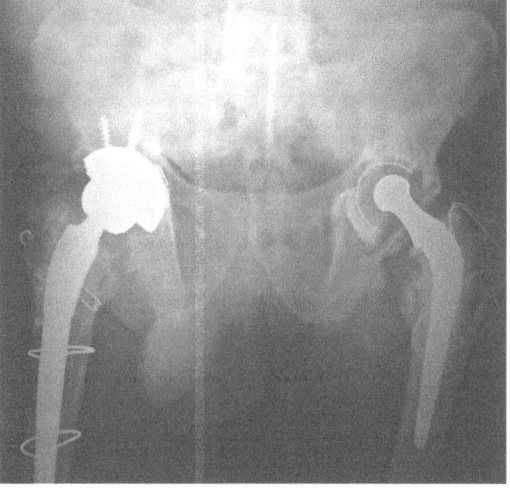

Fig. 1.25 Radiographs taken 37 years after primary
replacement of the left hip and 5 years after revision of the
right hip

1.6   Case 6

This female patient was born in 1928. Symptoms of the left hip started, because of eccentric idiopathic OA, around the age of 48 years. LFA was performed in 1980, when the patient was 52 years old. Early postoperative development of Brooker grade 2/3 heterotopic ossification, without any clinical effect, was developed. At the last clinical and radiographic evaluation, 35 years postoperatively, the patient was 87 years old, remained symptoms-free and had normal activity level (Figs. 1.26–1.29).

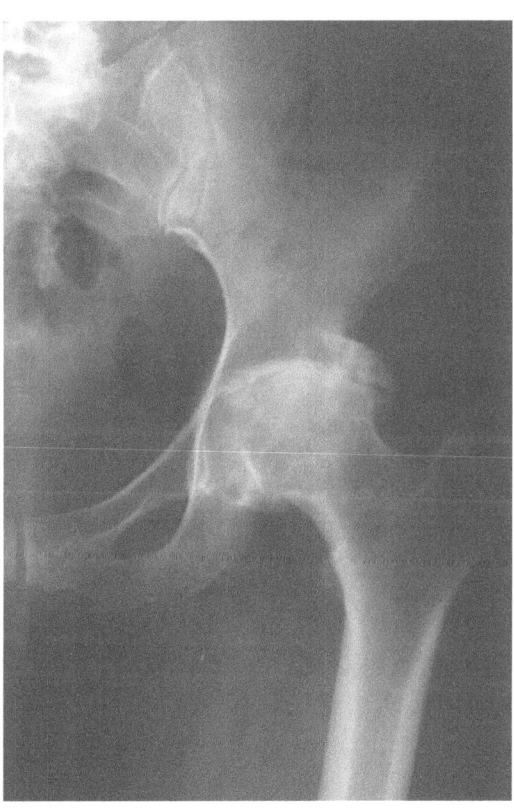

Fig. 1.26 Preoperative radiograph taken in 1980, when the patient was 52 years old

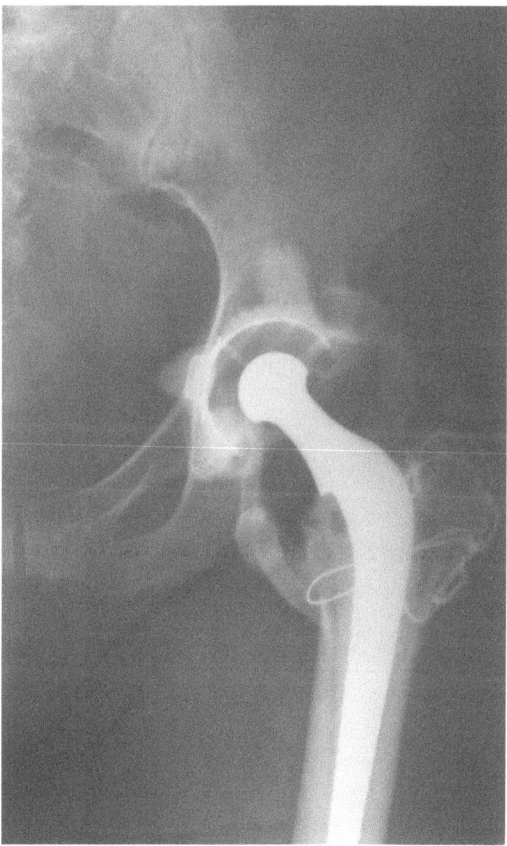

Fig. 1.27 Five years postoperatively, a Brooker grade 2/3 heterotopic ossification had been developed without any clinical impact

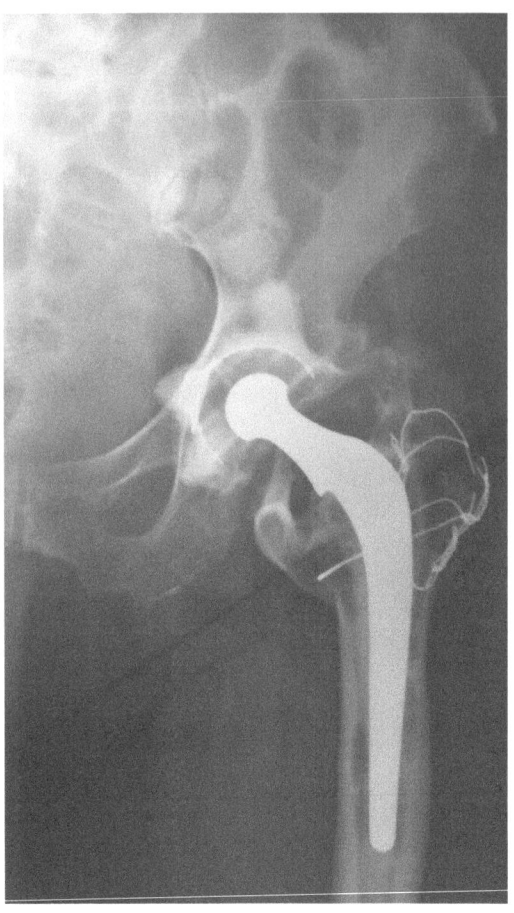

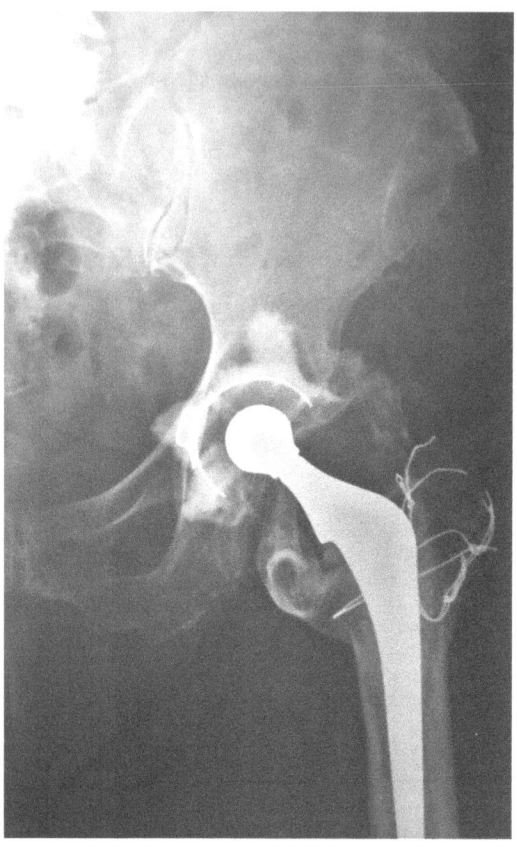

Fig. 1.29 The last postoperative radiograph taken 35 years after primary replacement

Fig. 1.28 Thirty years postoperatively

1.7 Case 7

This female patient was born in 1935. Symptoms of the left hip started, around the age of 43 years, because of eccentric idiopathic OA. LFA was performed when the patient was 46 years old, in 1981. Right hip also developed eccentric idiopathic OA many years later, and the patient had a THR in another institution in 2014, when she was 79 years old. Two years later, at the last follow-up examination, patient had no hip pain, retaining acceptable activity level (Figs. 1.30–1.34).

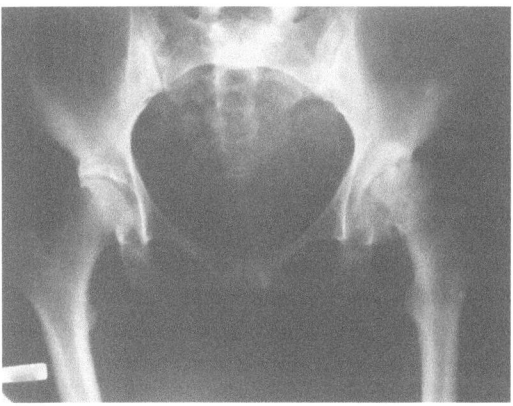

Fig. 1.30 Radiograph taken in 1981 when the patient was 46 years old and diagnosed with eccentric OA of the left hip. Right hip was normal. LFA was followed

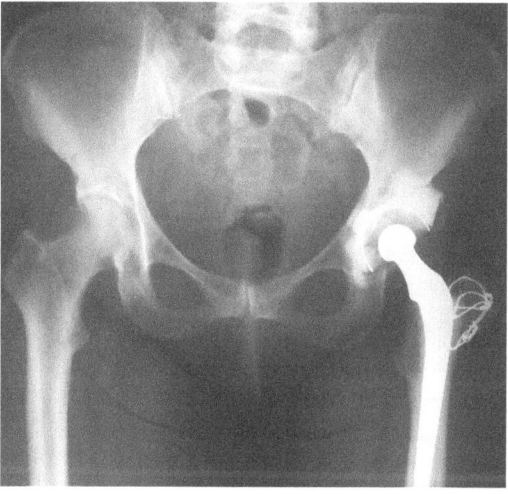

Fig. 1.32 At the 12th postoperative year of the left LFA. The right hip remained normal

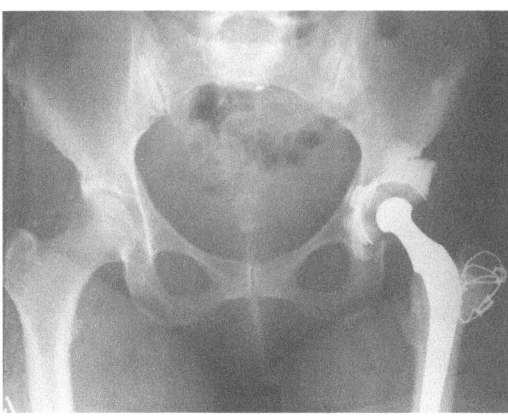

Fig. 1.31 One year after LFA of the left hip

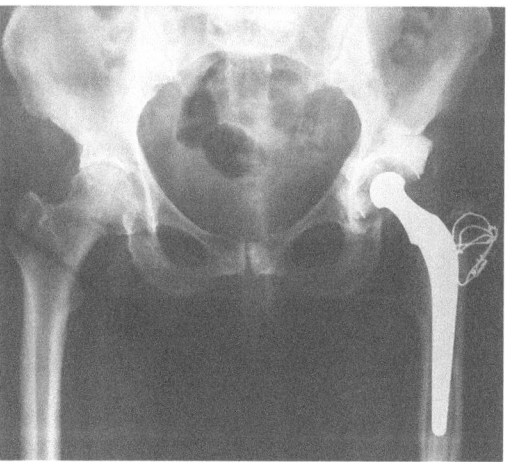

Fig. 1.33 Radiograph taken 27 years after replacement of the left hip. Both components were characterised as possibly loose. However, patient remained asymptomatic from the left hip and had mild pain in the right hip because of the onset of degenerative changes

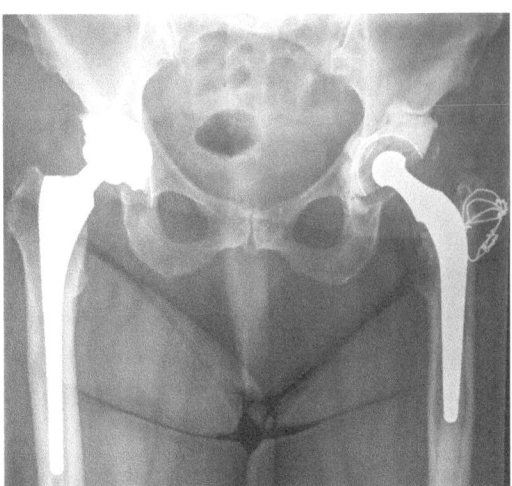

Fig. 1.34 At the latest radiograph follow-up evaluation, 35 years after LFA of the left hip and 2 years after uncemented THR of the right. Components of the left hip remained possibly loose without further progression of radiolucency

1.8   Case 8

This female patient was born in 1922. She had a limp on the left hip since infancy. She started complaining of pain around the age of 40 years. We examined her in 1975, when she was 53 years old. The diagnosis was secondary OA of the left hip because of low dislocation. She was limping heavily and had severe pain. LFA was performed. This was the only case of our registry that trochanteric osteotomy was not used. She had an uneventful postoperative course, and only a slight Trendelenburg gait remained.

At the age of 67 years, she started having pain in the right hip because of eccentric idiopathic OA. Two years later, in 1991, LFA was followed. At the last follow-up, 41 and 25 years after LFA of the left and right hip, respectively, the patient was 94 years old, and she had no hip pain and remained with an activity level compatible to her age (Figs. 1.35–1.38).

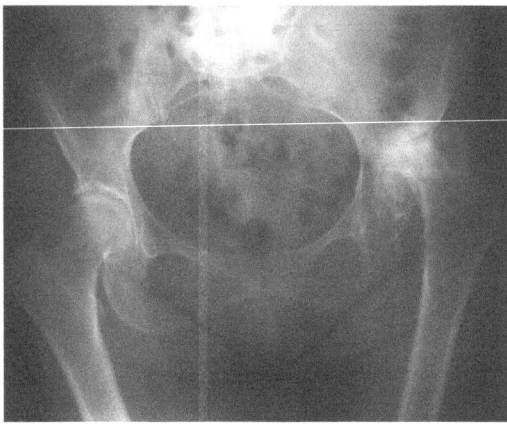

Fig. 1.35 Radiograph taken in 1975. The left hip had secondary OA because of low dislocation and the right was normal. LFA of the left hip was followed

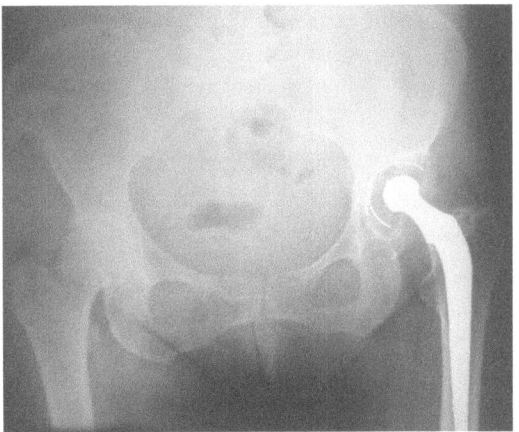

Fig. 1.36 Five years after LFA of the left hip. Note that the cup was placed in a high position and the stem, a round-back design, in a slight varus position. The cement is not visible on the radiograph because it did not contain barium

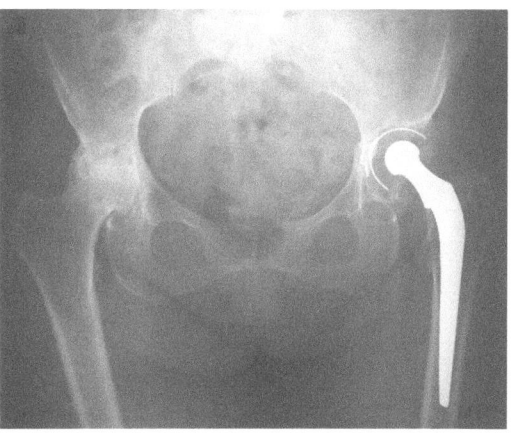

Fig. 1.37 Sixteen years after left THR, in 1991, the right hip had developed eccentric idiopathic OA. LFA was followed

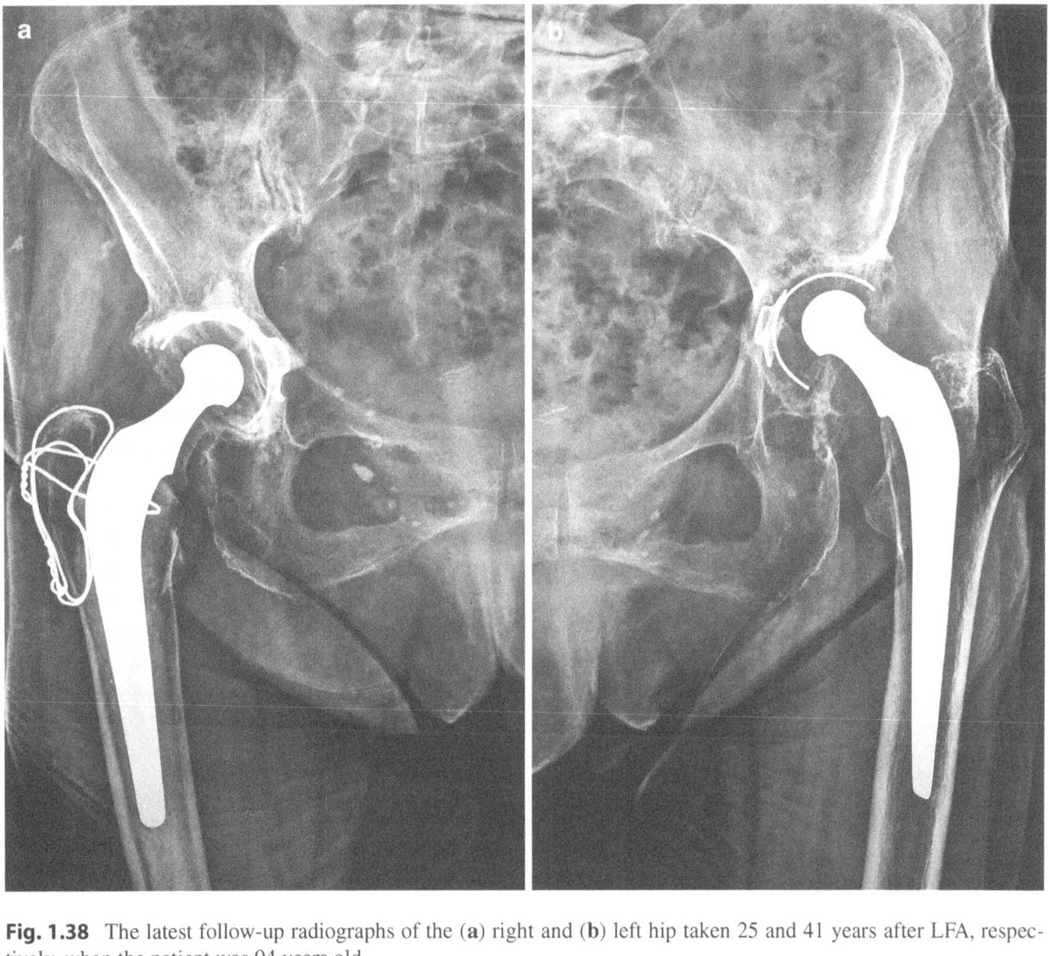

Fig. 1.38 The latest follow-up radiographs of the (**a**) right and (**b**) left hip taken 25 and 41 years after LFA, respectively, when the patient was 94 years old

1.9   Case 9

This female patient was born in 1950, and she had complete dislocation of the right hip. At the age of 3 years, she was operated (we have no information about the type of operation). She was limping since then, and around the age of 25 years, she started having pain. In 1980, when she was 30 years old, we performed an LFA. Approximately 8 years later, she started having slight pain and limping on the left hip, which radiographically was classified as dysplastic, with an early stage OA. The deterioration was slow, and THR was needed in this hip in 2001, when the patient was 51 years old. At the age of 66 years, when she had her last follow-up evaluation, she remained asymptomatic retaining normal activities, 36 and 15 years after THR of the right and the left hip, respectively (Figs. 1.39–1.43).

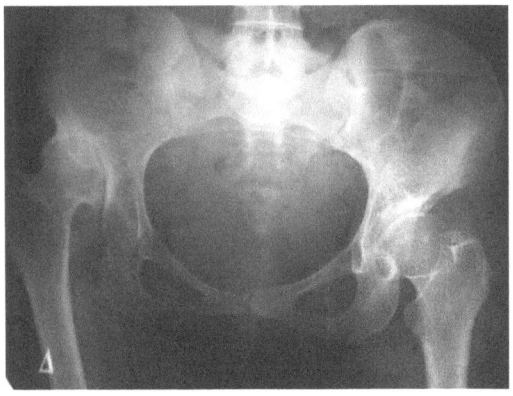

Fig. 1.39 Radiograph, when the patient was 30 years old, depicted high dislocation of the right hip and dysplasia of the left hip with an early stage OA. The left hip was asymptomatic

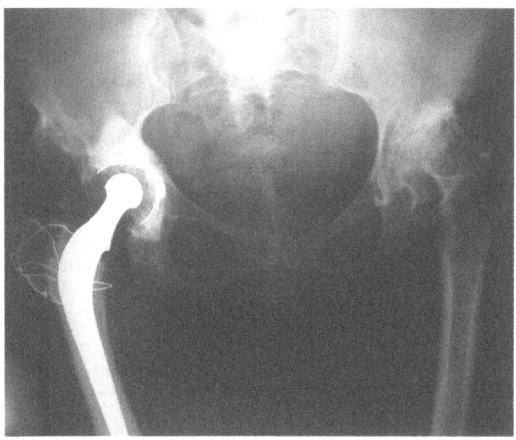

Fig. 1.41 Twenty years after LFA of the right hip in 2001. Further worsening of the left hip led to a THR

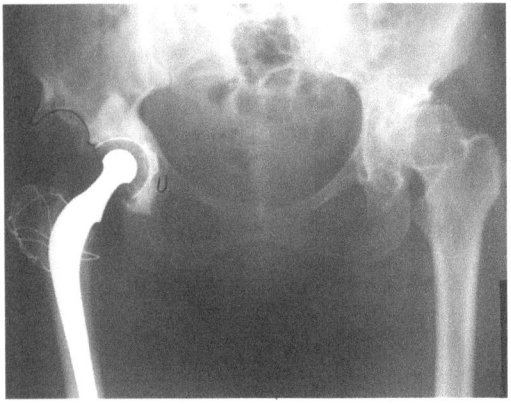

Fig. 1.40 Ten years after LFA of the right hip. Left hip presented deterioration of OA. Symptoms of this hip had started 2 years previously

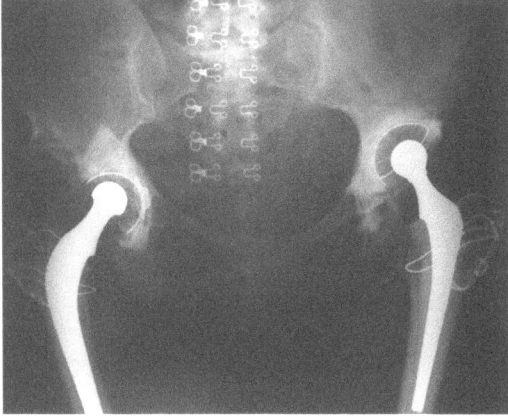

Fig. 1.42 Radiograph taken 28 years after THR of the right hip and 7 years of the left

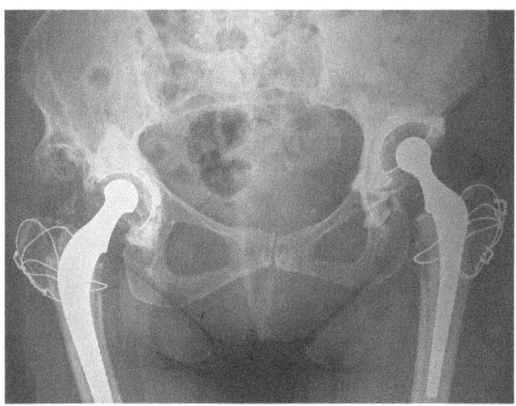

Fig. 1.43 The latest follow-up radiograph, 36 and 15 years after right and left THR, respectively. Wear of the right acetabular component was not associated with notable osteolysis. Further observation was suggested

1.10   Case 10

This female patient was born in 1929. She began to have pain from the left hip, because of the development of eccentric idiopathic OA, around the age of 45 years. At the age of 52 years, in 1981, an LFA was performed. At the 15-year follow-up examination, both components were classified as probably loose; however, they did not present any worsening over the following 20 years, since the latest follow-up examination, performed 35 years after initial operation. At the age of 87 years, the patient remains asymptomatic with an activity level compatible to her age (Figs. 1.44–1.49).

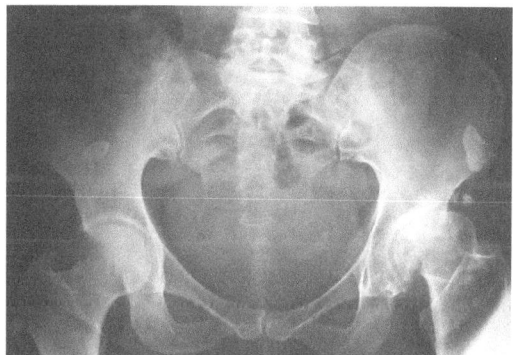

Fig. 1.44 Preoperative radiograph in 1981, when the patient was 52 years old

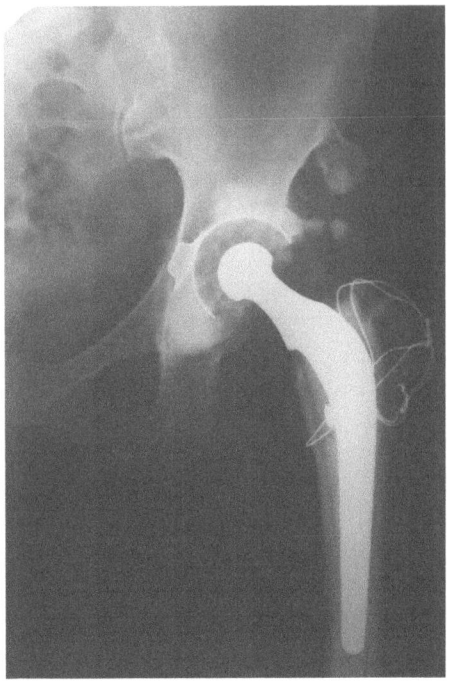

Fig. 1.45 Early postoperative radiograph. Note the improper distribution of the cement around the acetabular component

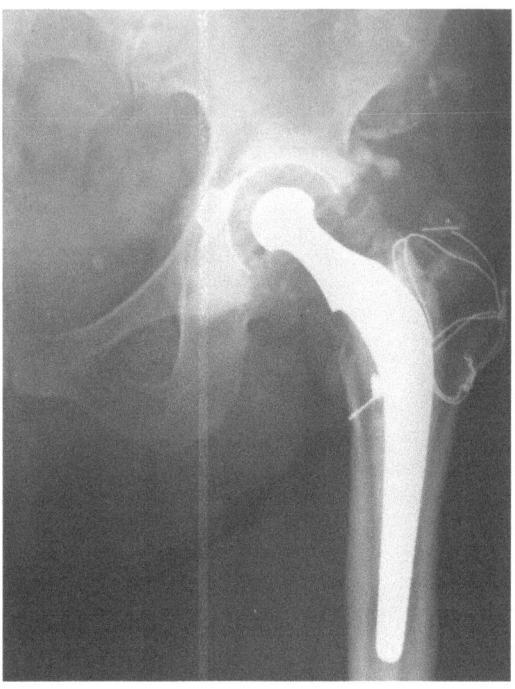

Fig. 1.47 Fifteen years postoperatively. Both components were considered probably loose

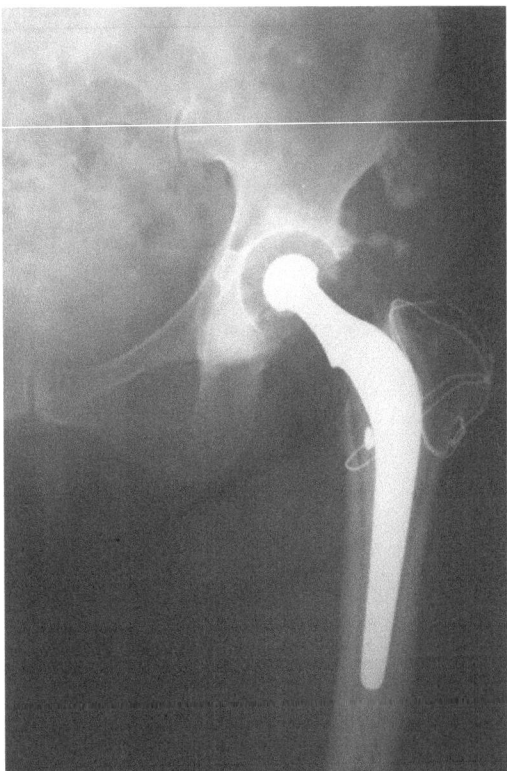

Fig. 1.46 Radiograph taken 5 years after surgery. Both components were classified as well-fixed

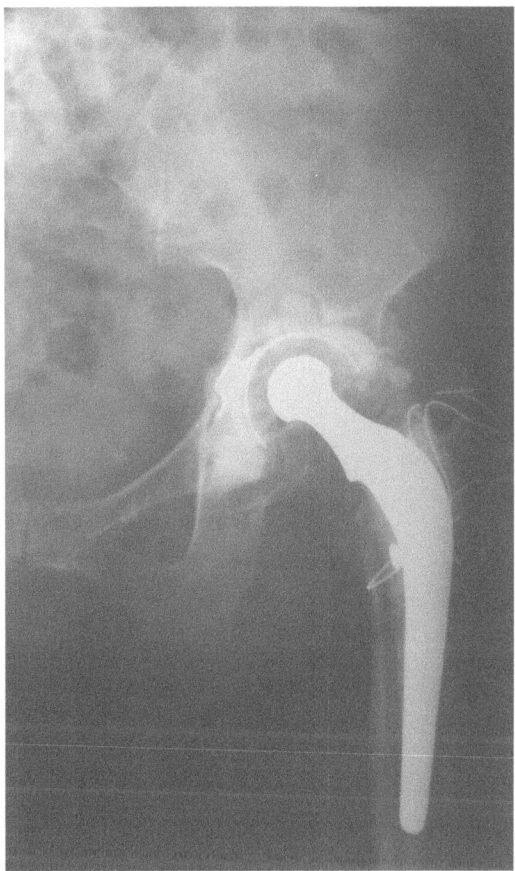

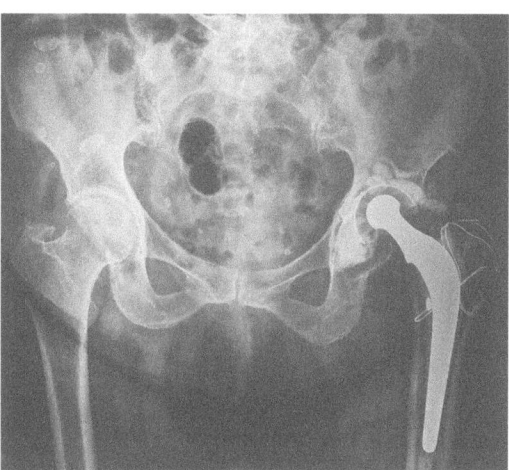

Fig. 1.49 The latest follow-up radiograph taken 35 years after THR, when the patient was 87 years old. Although both components were classified as probably loose for more than 20 years, they had not presented any migration

Fig. 1.48 Twenty-eight years postoperatively. Both components remained in place with a slight further deterioration

Late treatment with closed reduction and prolonged plaster immobilisation in extreme abduction of newborns with CHD, was the common practice in earlier decades. As a result, the disordered anatomy of these hips made a future THR technically even more difficult. This situation significantly improved over time with the introduction of the use of ultrasound as a screening test and early application of a proper treatment. Consequently, in recent years, orthopaedic surgeons rather seldom come up against patients with severe hip deformities because of late treatment in infancy.

Our registry includes many cases presenting disappointing results of late closed reduction and prolonged immobilisation with plaster. We present these cases for historical reason and for examples to avoid.

2.1 Case 1

This female patient was born in 1948 with congenital disease of both hips. At the age of 4 years, she was treated by her physician with closed reduction and immobilisation in hip spica for more than 2 years, followed by open reduction of the left hip. A major disability remained with heavy limping and severe leg-length discrepancy. We examined the patient, at the age of 38 years, in 1986. Her right hip was classified as having dysplasia and her left low dislocation. She was 135 cm tall, and the left leg had 11 cm shortening. LFA was performed, first in the right hip and within 5 weeks in the left. Leg-length discrepancy was decreased to 7 cm.

Since then, patient had a better quality of life for many years. However, revision, because of aseptic loosening of implants of both hips, was needed, in 2005, 19 years after primary replacements. The revision of the right hip was complicated with a periprosthetic fracture, 4 months later, and this was treated with internal fixation.

At the latest follow-up, 30 years after primary procedures, and 11 years after the revision of both hips, the patient although was limping had no hip pain and reported fair quality of life (Figs. 2.1–2.8).

© Springer International Publishing AG 2017
K. Lampropoulou-Adamidou, G. Hartofilakidis, *Total Hip Replacement*,
DOI 10.1007/978-3-319-53360-5_2

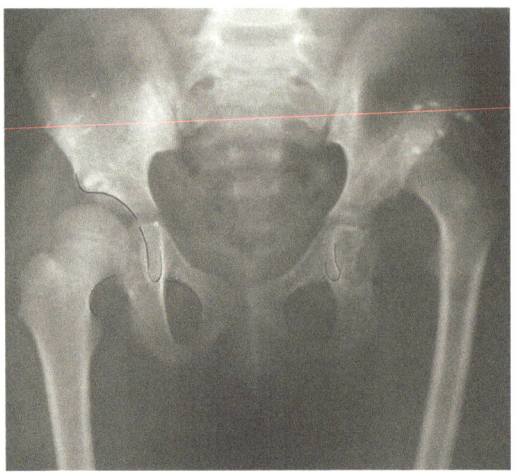

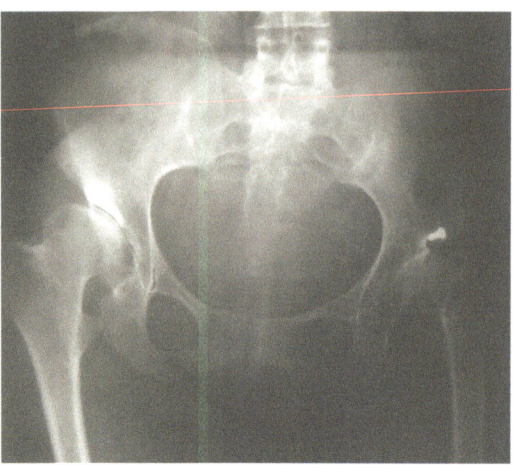

Fig. 2.1 Radiograph, taken at the age of 6 years, during conservative treatment and before the attempt of open reduction of the left hip

Fig 2.2 At the age of 28 years, radiograph presented dysplastic right hip and left hip with low dislocation

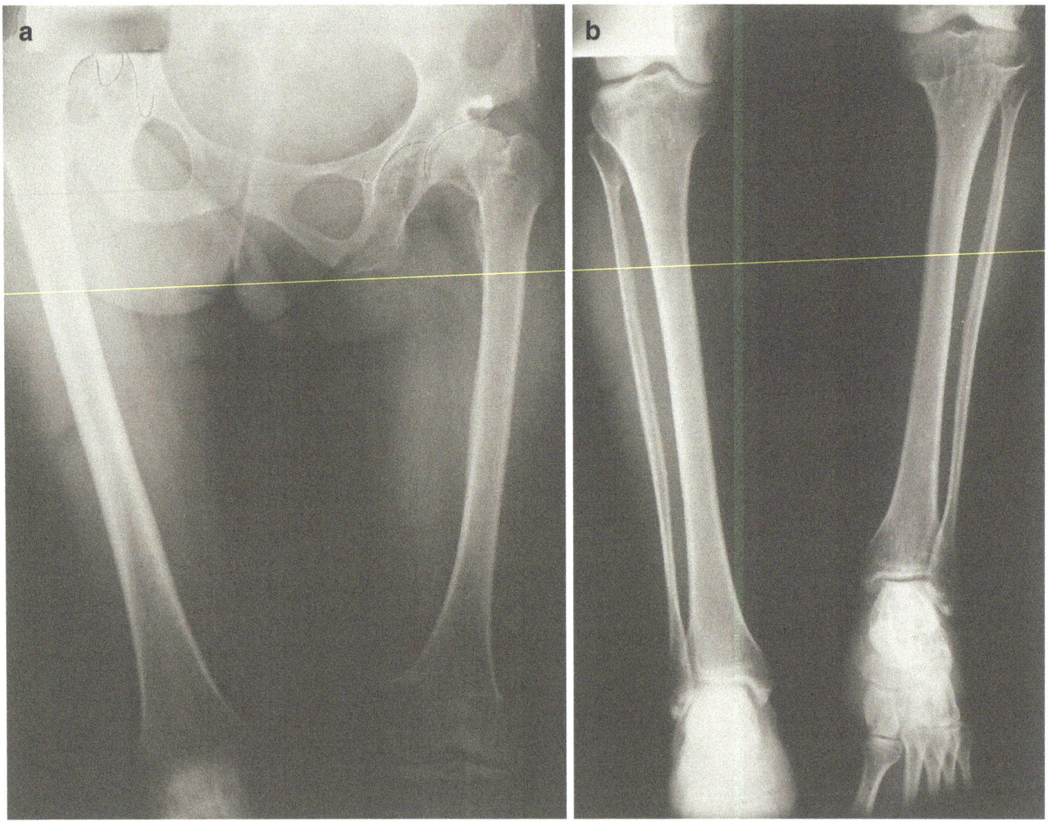

Fig. 2.3 At the age of 38 years, when the patient was referred to us in 1986. Radiographs of (**a**) both hips and femurs and (**b**) both tibia. Note the severe leg-length discrepancy. THR of both hips was followed

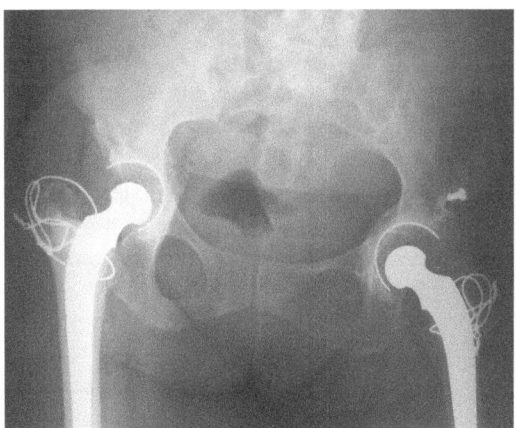

Fig. 2.4 One year after LFA of both hips

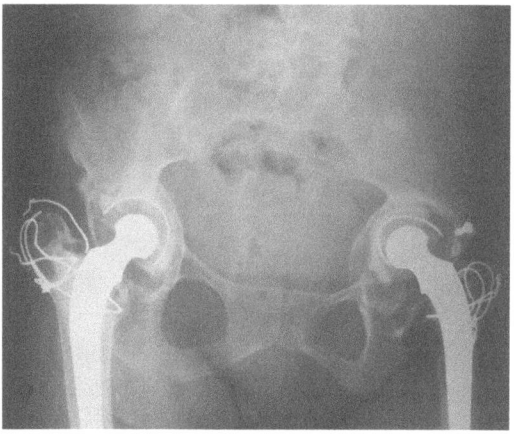

Fig. 2.6 Nineteen years postoperatively in 2005. Both acetabular components were loose and needed to be revised. Her surgeon decided to revise both components of both hips within 3 months

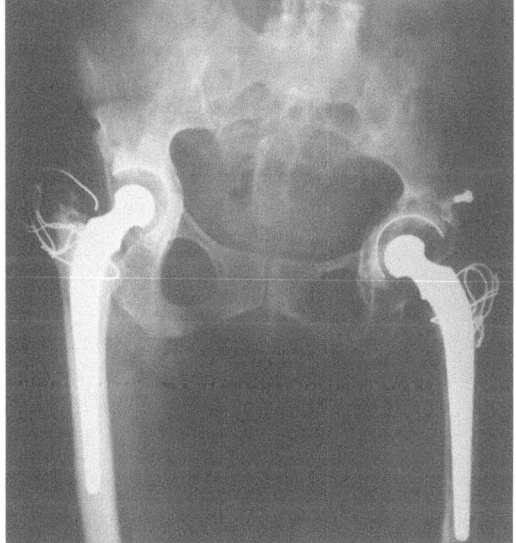

Fig. 2.5 Ten years postoperatively

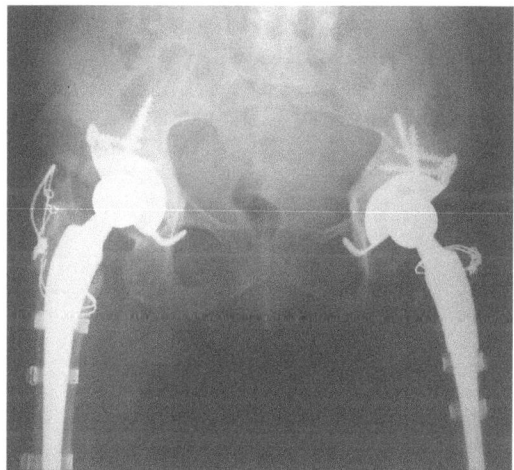

Fig. 2.7 Two months after revision

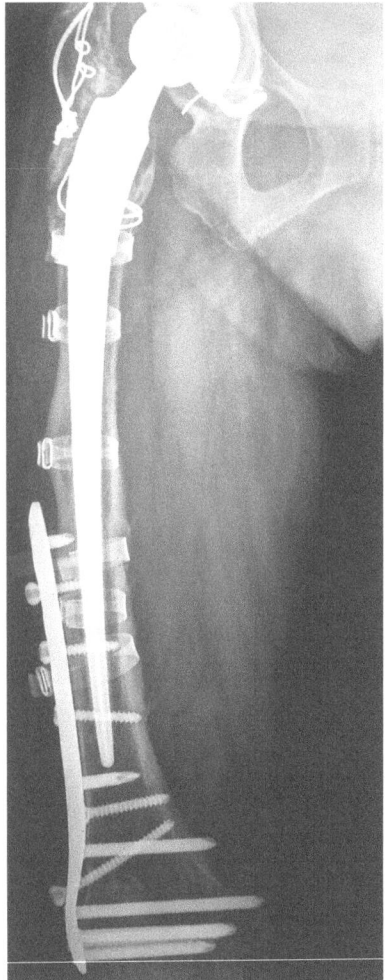

Fig. 2.8 A periprosthetic fracture of the right femur occurred 4 months after revision, treated with open reduction and internal fixation. This radiograph was taken 7 years after the latest procedure and 26 years after the primary THRs

2.2   Case 2

This female patient was born in 1966 with complete dislocation of both hips. At the age of 2 years, she was treated by her physician with closed reduction and prolonged immobilisation in hip spica, followed by open reduction of both hips, 1 year later. She was limping since then and she started to have pain around the age of 20 years. We examined her when she was 29 years old. She was limping heavily and had severe hip pain and disability. We performed hybrid THR in both hips in 1995. Revision of polyethylene liner and stem of the left and right hip 14 and 15 years after primary THRs, respectively, was performed by one of the members of our team.

At the latest follow-up evaluation, 21 years after primary replacements and 6 and 7 years after the revision of the right and left hip, respectively, the patient was fully active and had no pain although she was walking with bilateral Trendelenburg gait (Figs. 2.9–2.18).

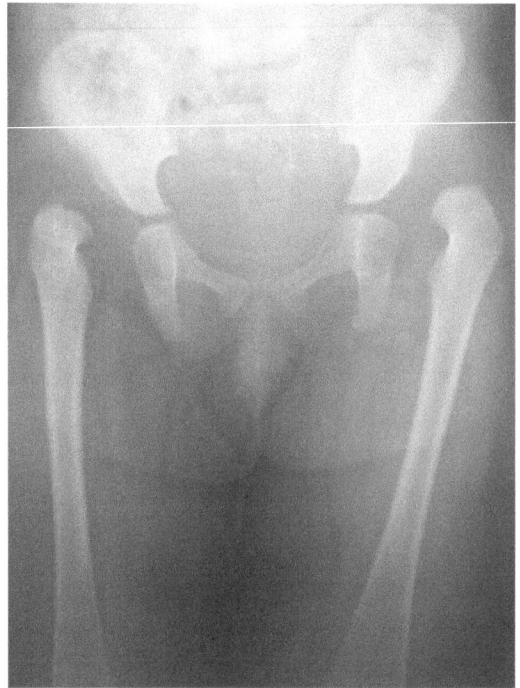

Fig. 2.9 Radiograph before any treatment, when the patient was 2 years old

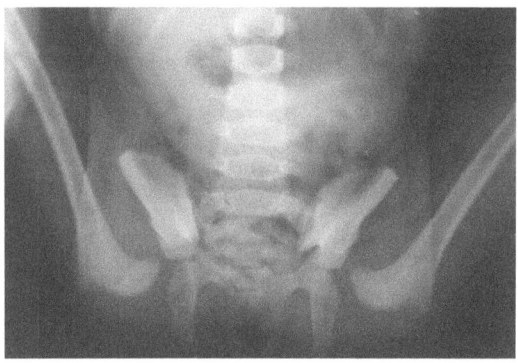

Fig. 2.10 Radiograph of 1968 with the hips in extreme abduction in a hip spica after closed reduction

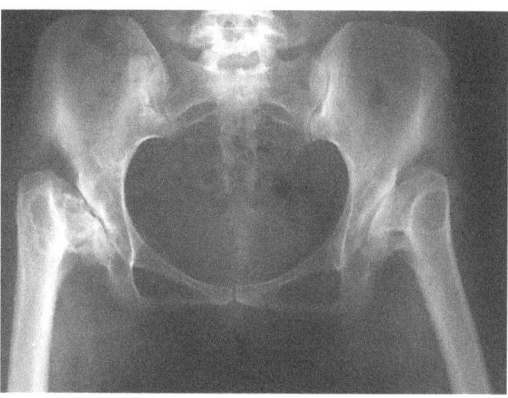

Fig. 2.13 Radiograph when we first examined her in 1995, at the age of 29 years

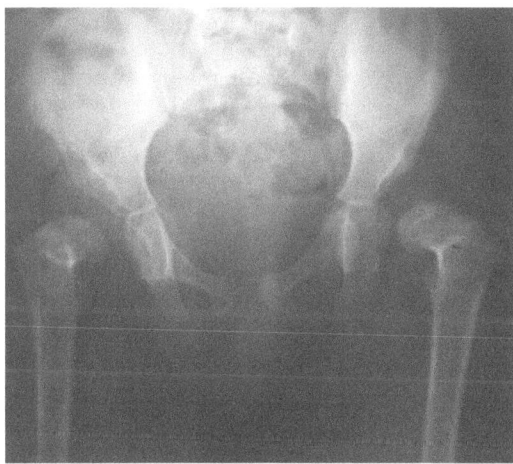

Fig. 2.11 At the age of 3 years, after open reduction of both hips. There is a remarkable damage to the ossification centre of the femoral heads

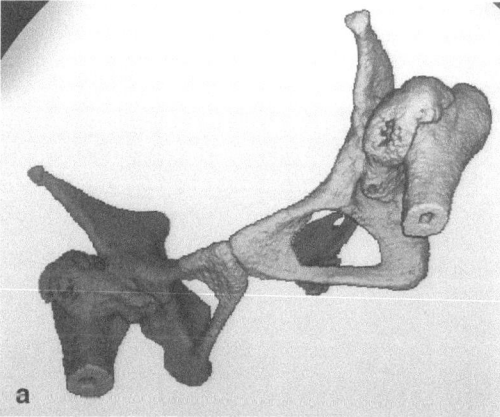

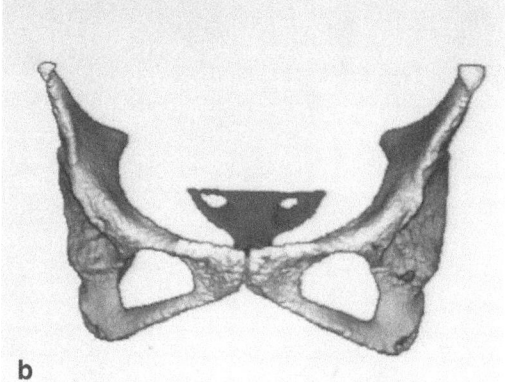

Fig. 2.14 Preoperative assessment with 3D CT scans (**a**) with and (**b**) without the femoral heads. Note the severe damage to the acetabuli and the femoral heads

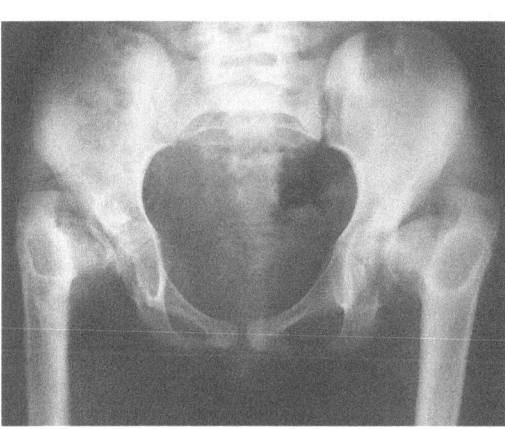

Fig. 2.12 Radiograph made when she was 12 years old

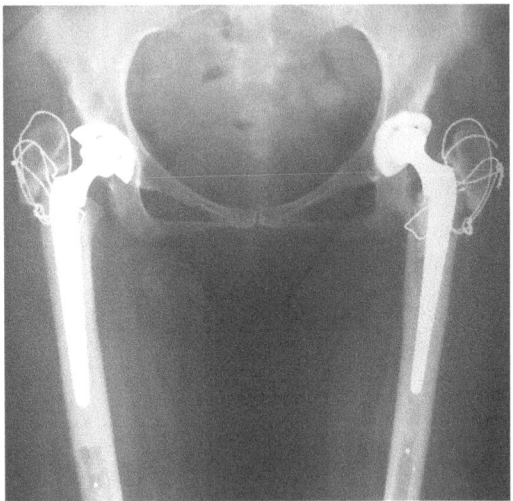

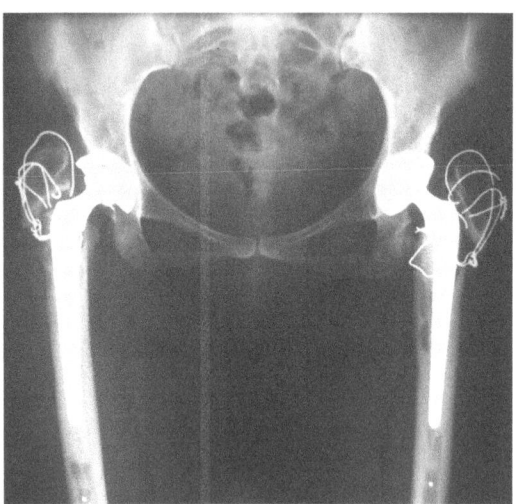

Fig. 2.15 Postoperative radiograph. Hybrid THR was performed in both hips

Fig. 2.16 Seven years postoperatively

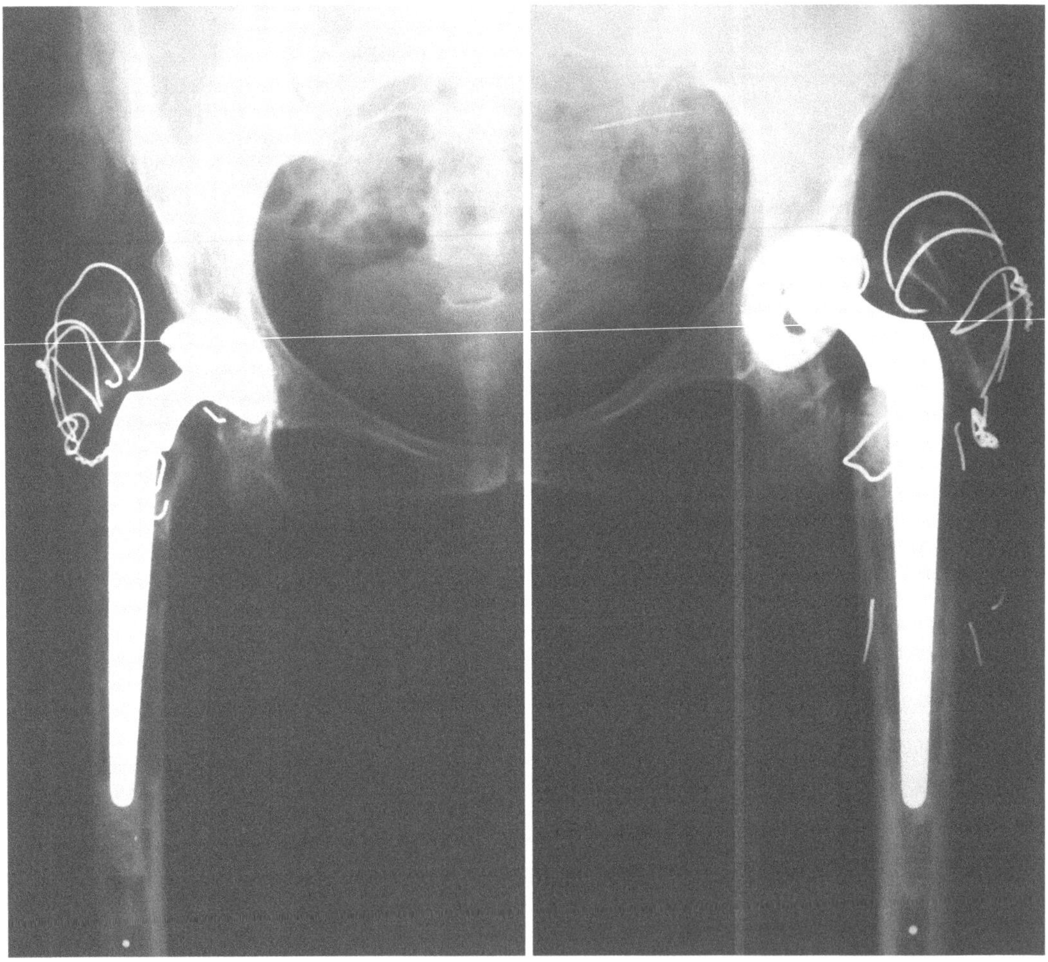

Fig. 2.17 Radiograph taken 14 years after primary replacements. Polyethylene liner wear of both hips, more pronounced in the left hip, is obvious. Revision of polyethylene and stem of the left and right hip was followed

Fig. 2.18 The last follow-up radiograph of the (**a**) right and (**b**) left hip was taken 21 years after primary replacements and 6 and 7 years after revision of the right and left hip, respectively

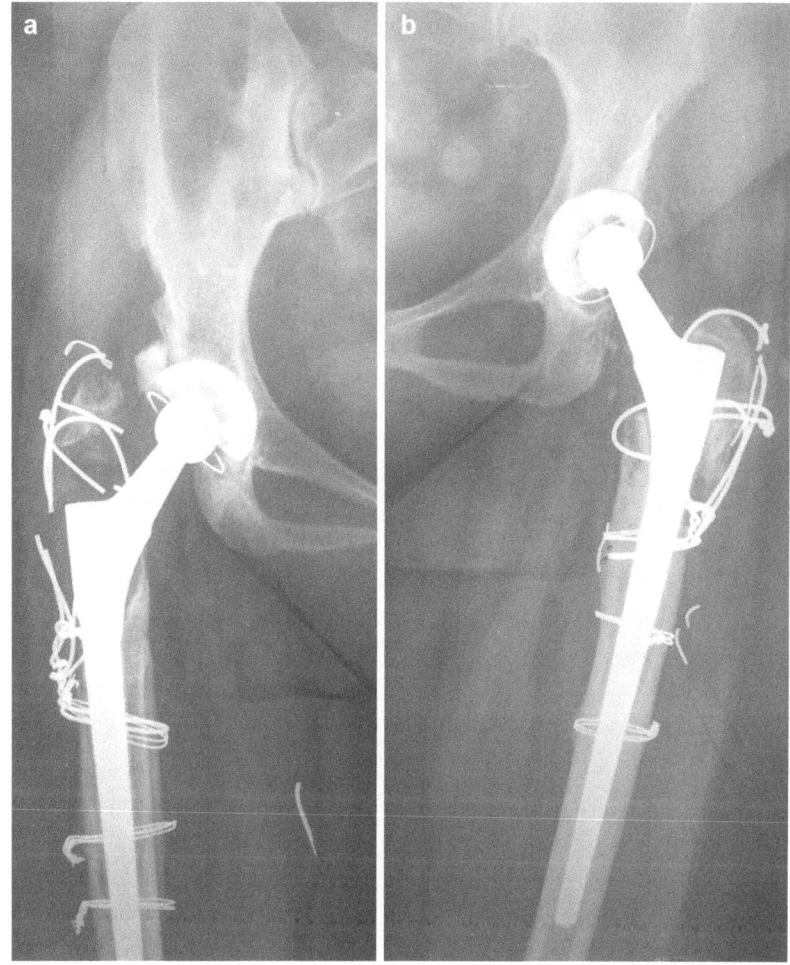

2.3   Case 3

This female patient was born in 1955. At the age of 2 years, she was treated by her physician with closed reduction and prolonged immobilisation in plaster for subluxation of the left hip. She was limping since infancy. At the age of 14 years, she underwent a subtrochanteric osteotomy by the same physician. Around the age of 30 years, she started having left hip pain. We examined her when she was 38 years old in 1993. A hybrid THR was performed. Preoperative assessment, using 3D CT scan, confirmed the evolution of subluxation to low dislocation.

Twenty-three years after THR, the patient, at the age of 61 years, remained without hip pain or limping and has normal activity level (Figs. 2.19–2.25).

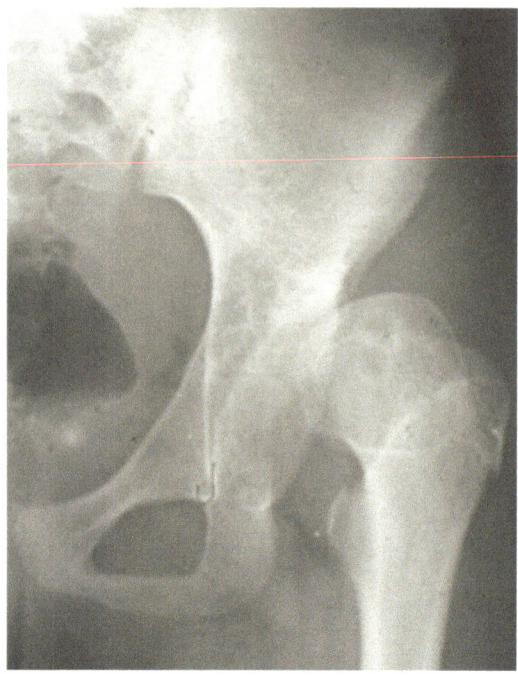

Fig. 2.20 At the age of 12 years, radiograph confirmed that the hip was not reduced by the previous treatment

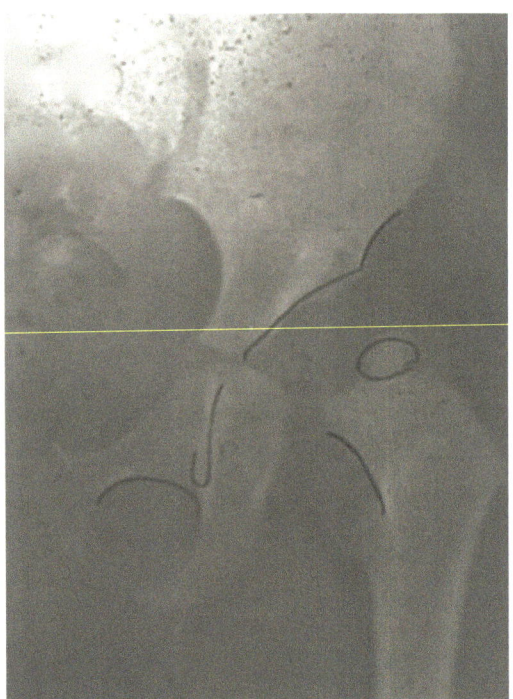

Fig. 2.19 Radiograph of the left hip before any treatment, when the patient was 2 years old. The subluxation is easily recognised

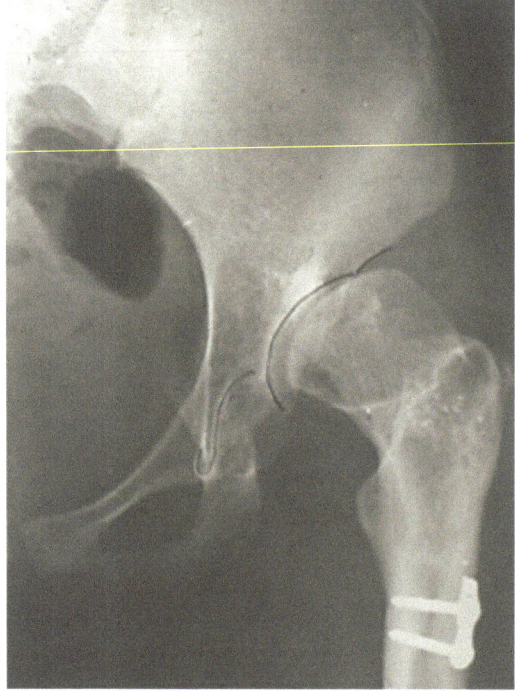

Fig. 2.21 At the age of 16 years, after the subtrochanteric osteotomy. A false acetabulum had started to develop

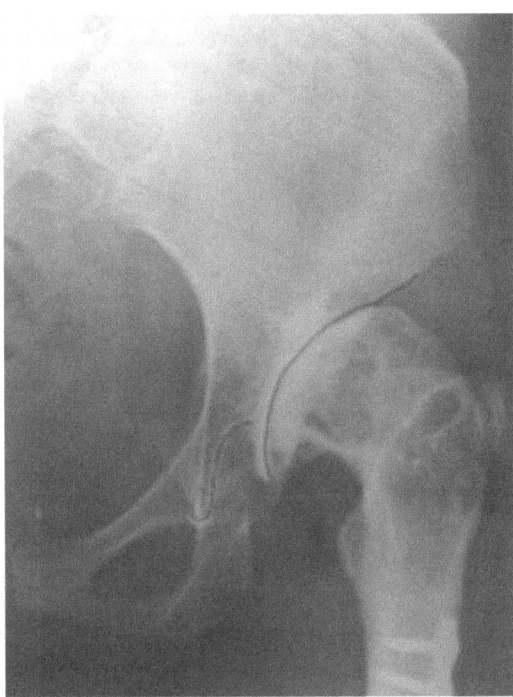

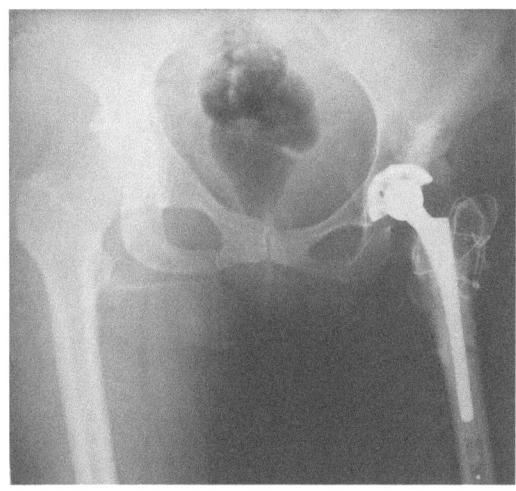

Fig. 2.24 Postoperative radiograph

Fig 2.22 Preoperative radiograph, when the patient was 37 years old and had a well-established low dislocation

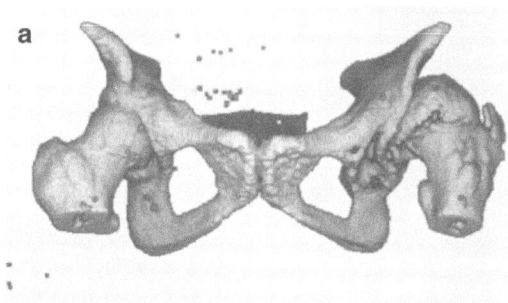

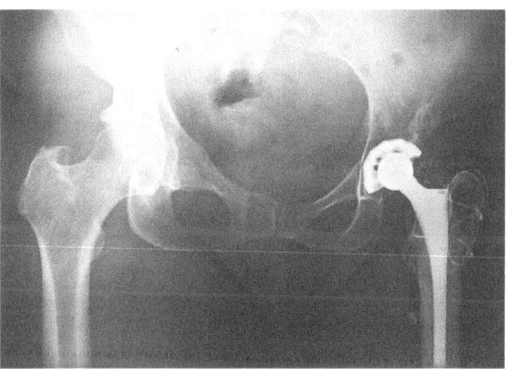

Fig. 2.25 The latest follow-up radiograph, 23 years postoperatively

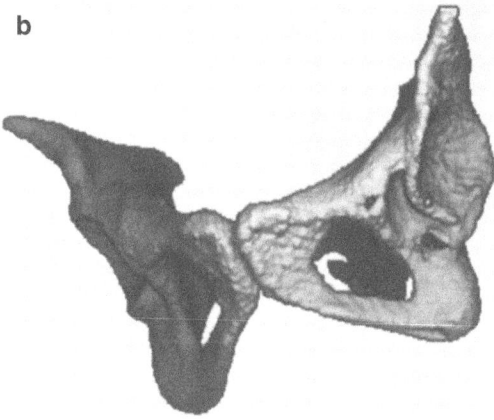

Fig. 2.23 Preoperative assessment with 3D CT scan (**a**) with and (**b**) without femoral head confirmed the diagnosis of B1 subtype low dislocation and facilitated our preoperative planning

2.4   Case 4

This female patient was born in 1949 with bilateral CHD. At the age of 18 months, her physician treated her with closed reduction and immobilisation in plaster. Ever since then, she was limping. Around the age of 20 years, pain in both hips started with slow deterioration during the next years. At the age of 42 years, in 1991, we operated her in both hips within 20 days. Both hips were classified as dysplastic. At the most recent follow-up examination, 25 years postoperatively, at the age of 67 years, she had no pain and no limp, and she was retaining a normal activity level (Figs. 2.26–2.29).

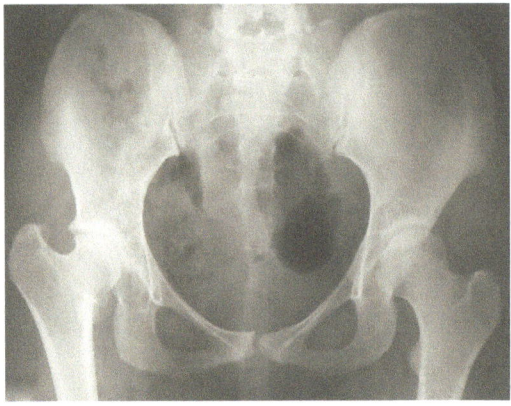

Fig. 2.26   At the age of 19 years, radiograph depicts bilateral dysplastic hips

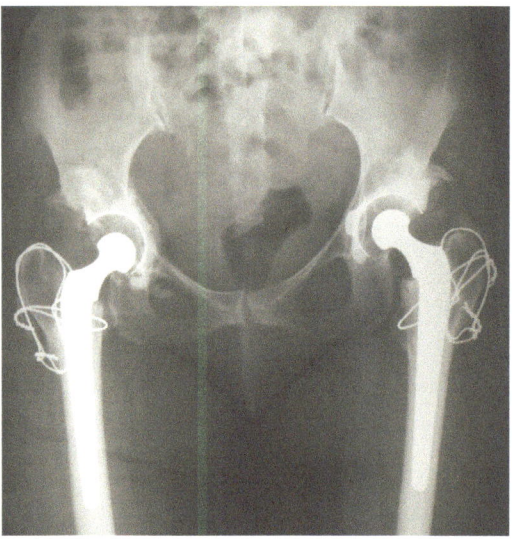

Fig. 2.28   Postoperative radiograph. In the right hip, offset-bore acetabulum with cotyloplasty was used

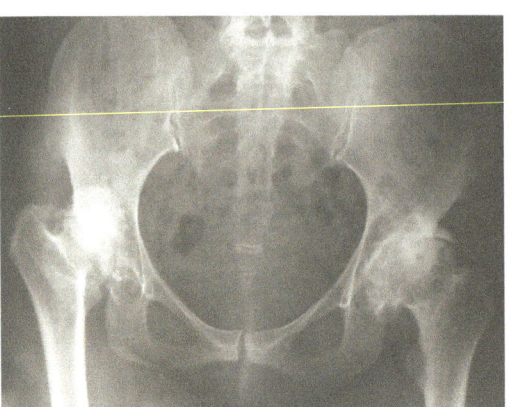

Fig. 2.27   At the age of 42 years, in 1991, when LFA of both hips was performed

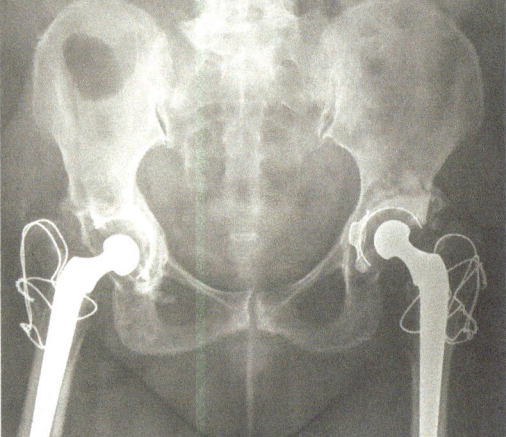

Fig. 2.29   The latest follow-up radiograph, 25 years postoperatively

2.5   Case 5

This female patient was born in 1939 with CHD of the right hip. Closed reduction attempted by her physician, when she was 4 years old, led to an unsuccessful result, with necrosis of the femoral head and a great deformity of the joint. When we first examined the patient at the age of 39 years, in 1978, her right hip was classified as having low dislocation. An LFA was performed. After 18 years, in 1996, both components were revised because of aseptic loosening.

Meanwhile, at the age of 48 years, she started limping and having pain in the left hip, because of the development of idiopathic OA. She underwent LFA of the left hip, in 1990, when she was 51 years old.

At the latest follow-up evaluation, 20 years after the revision of the right hip and 26 years after primary THR of the left, the patient, at the age of 77, had a normal life without hip pain (Figs. 2.30–2.33).

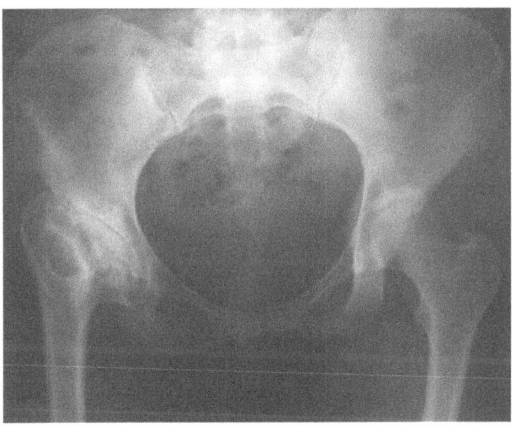

Fig. 2.30 Radiograph of the patient taken in 1978. The right hip was classified as having low dislocation. The left hip was normal

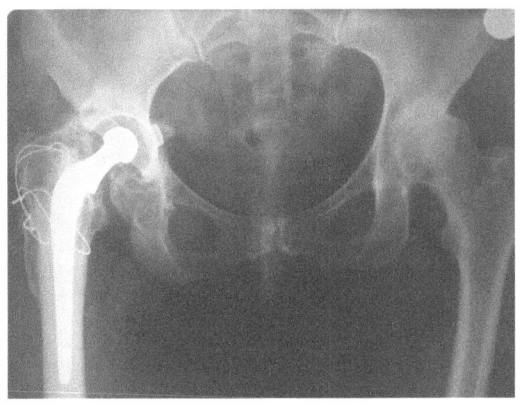

Fig. 2.31 Eleven years after LFA of the right hip. Left hip pain had started a year previously, because of the development of idiopathic eccentric OA

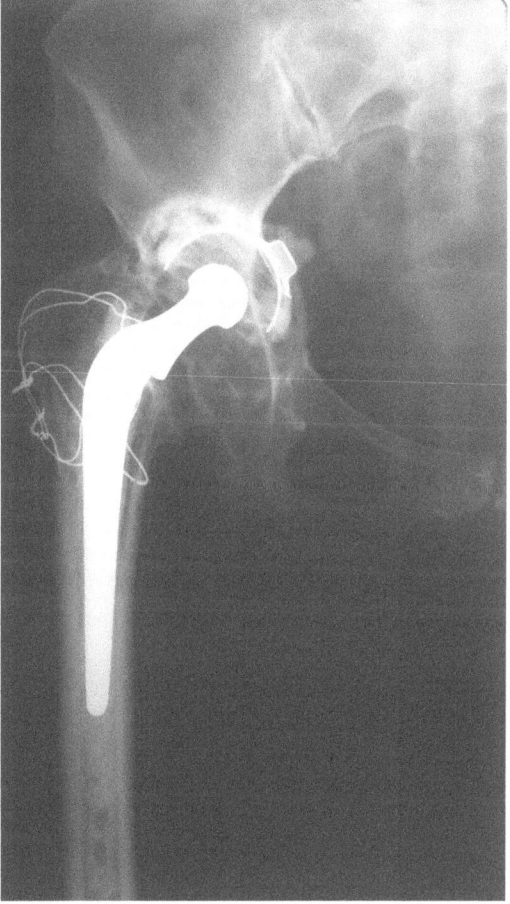

Fig. 2.32 Right acetabular component loosening and migration occurred 18 years after primary implantation. Revision of both components was followed

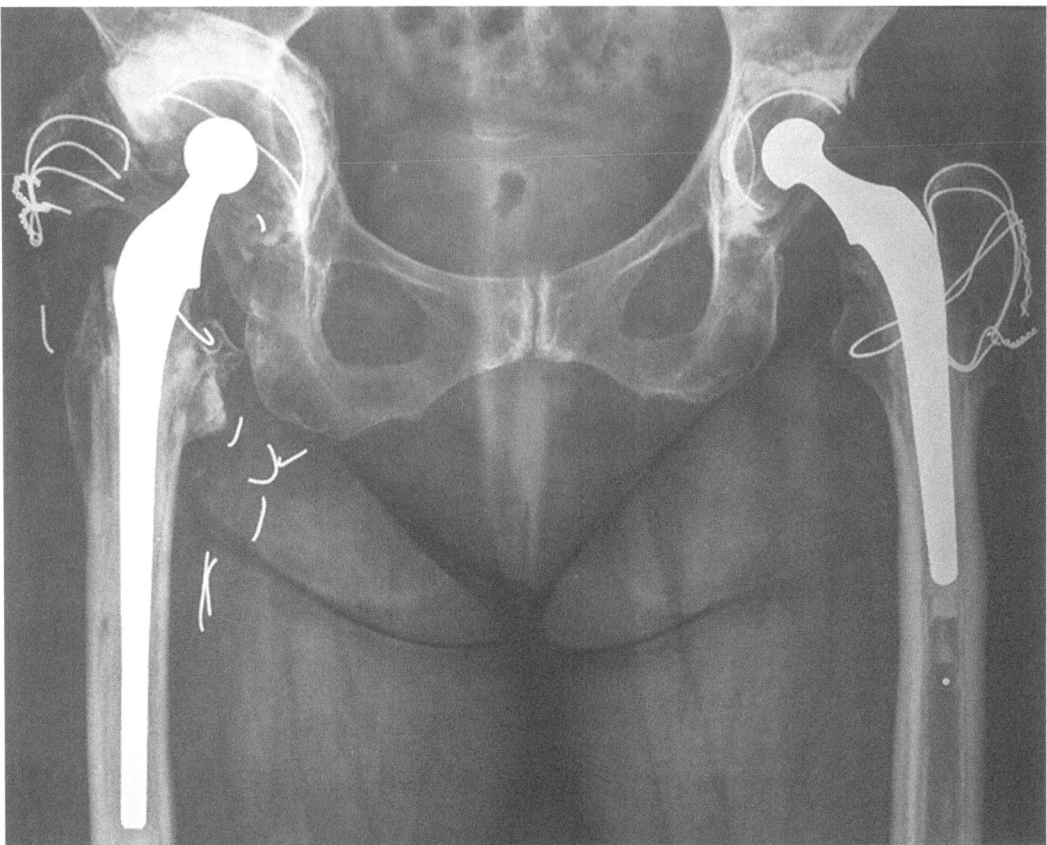

Fig. 2.33 The latest follow-up radiograph taken 20 years after the revision of the right hip and 26 years after primary replacement of the left hip

Before the introduction of THR, the treatment of choice in adults with CHD was intertrochanteric osteotomy. During these years, osteotomies were mostly performed without clear indication, and their results were not always satisfactory. The best results and the longest postponement of most radical procedures, such as THR, were obtained with the varus intertrochanteric osteotomy, in the early stages of the development of OA in dysplastic hips, and the valgus intertrochanteric osteotomy in a later stage. Recent years, osteotomies in adults with CHD are rarely performed. For that reason, surgeons usually have limited experience in this type of operations and should be decided with caution.

THR in patients with previous intertrochanteric osteotomies presents additional technical difficulties, especially when there is a major displacement. In cases where the implants of fixation of the previous osteotomy are still in place, we recommend a two-stage procedure: first, removal of the implants, and after 1–2 years, THR reconstruction.

3.1 Case 1

This female patient was born in 1939 with bilateral CHD. Her physician treated her, at the age of 3 years, with closed reduction and immobilisation in plaster. She was limping since infancy. Pain started around the age of 25 years and was more pronounced in the right hip. We examined the patient in 1970, when she was 31 years old. She had low dislocation of the right hip and high dislocation of the left. We performed a McMurray osteotomy of the right hip. A Wainwright plate was used for the fixation of osteotomy, which was removed 2 years later. Twenty-three years after osteotomy, in 1993, THR was necessary. The same year, a hybrid THR was performed in the left hip. The following years, she had, in another institution, three more operations: in 2005, 12 years after primary THR, revision of both components of the left hip because of aseptic loosening; in 2006, 13 years after primary THR, revision of both components of the right hip for the same reason; and in 2008, revision of the left cup also because of loosening.

The patient died from cardiac arrest, 40 days after the last operation at the age of 69 years (Figs. 3.1–3.6).

K. Lampropoulou-Adamidou, G. Hartofilakidis, *Total Hip Replacement*, DOI 10.1007/978-3-319-53360-5_3

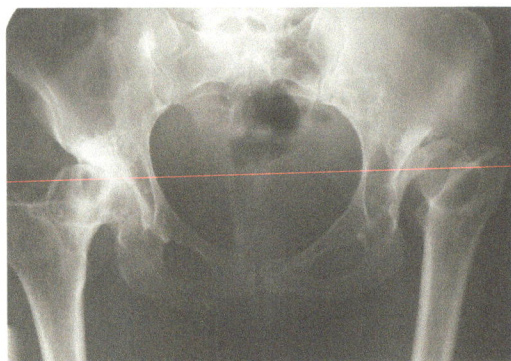

Fig. 3.1 Radiograph, when the patient was 31 years old, in 1970. She had low dislocation of the right hip and high dislocation of the left. A McMurray osteotomy of the right hip was followed

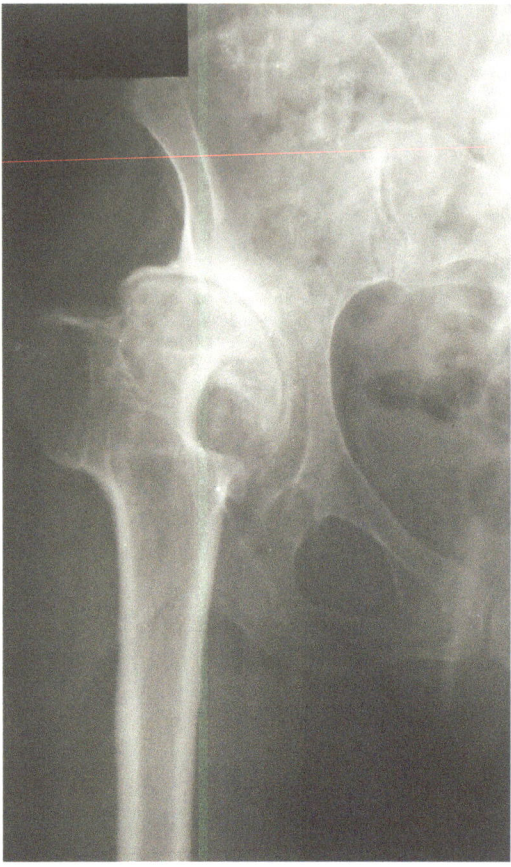

Fig. 3.3 Twenty-three years after osteotomy in 1993, when THR was decided

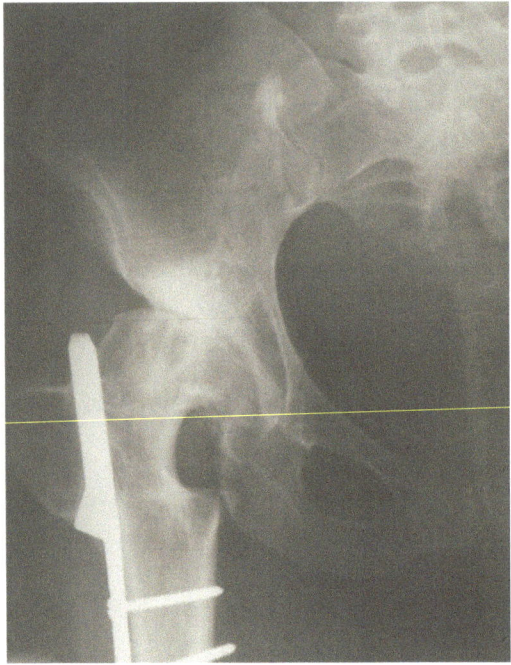

Fig. 3.2 One year after osteotomy. A Wainwright fixation plate was used that was removed after 2 years

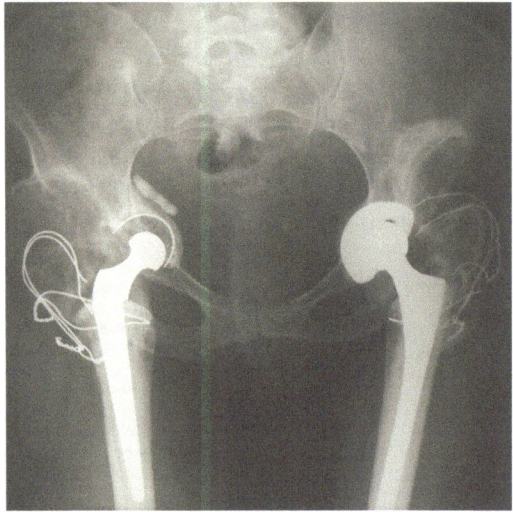

Fig. 3.4 Radiograph after LFA of the right hip and hybrid THR of the left

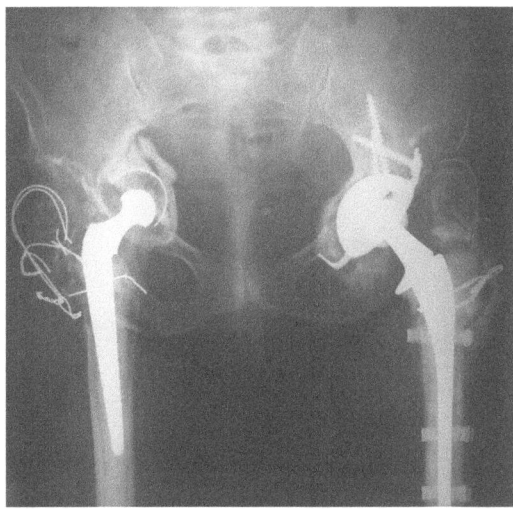

Fig. 3.5 Radiograph taken in 2006, 1 year after revision of both components of the left hip and 13 years after primary LFA of the right. Revision of both components of the right hip was followed

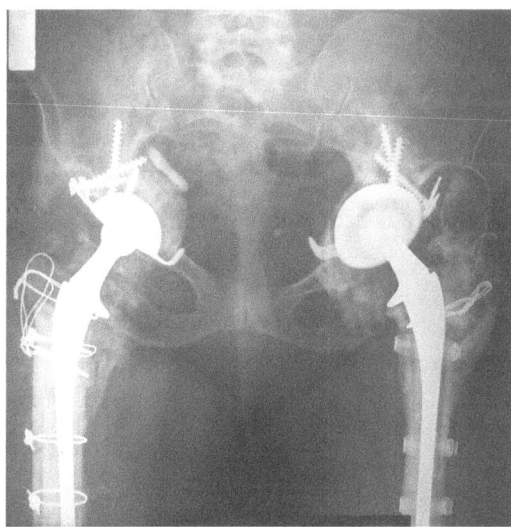

Fig. 3.6 Two years after revision of both components of the right hip and before the second revision of the cup only of the left. Forty days after the last operation, the patient died from cardiac arrest

3.2   Case 2

This female patient was born in 1952 with complete dislocation of the left hip. She was limping heavily since infancy and pain started around the age of 15 years. At the age of 18 years, she had by her physician a Schanz-type osteotomy. Seven years later, in 1977, when we first examined her, she had severe pain and great limitation of hip range of motion and she was limping heavily. We treated her with LFA. Thirty-nine years after THR, at the age of 64 years, the patient remained without pain in the left hip, although she was limping and had limited range of motion (Figs. 3.7–3.10).

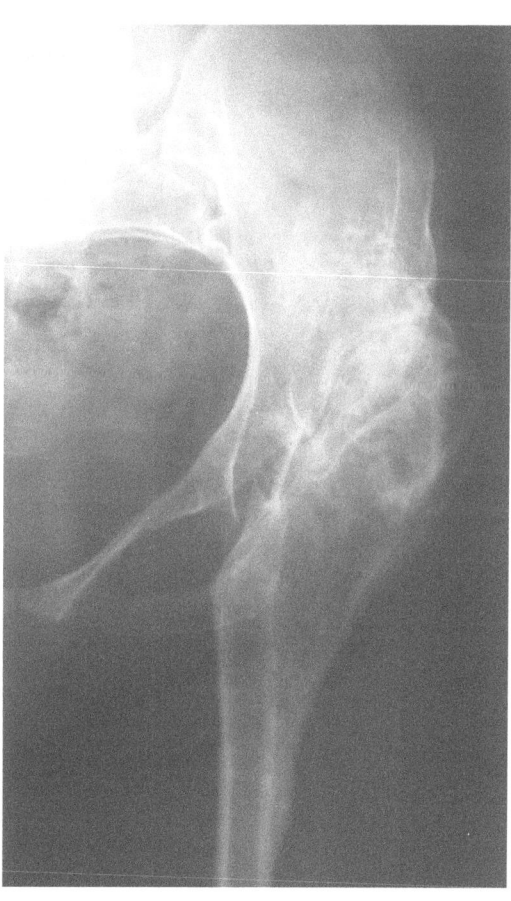

Fig. 3.7 Radiograph of the left hip taken in 1977, when the patient was 25 years old. She had high dislocation with a previous Schanz osteotomy. A THR was followed

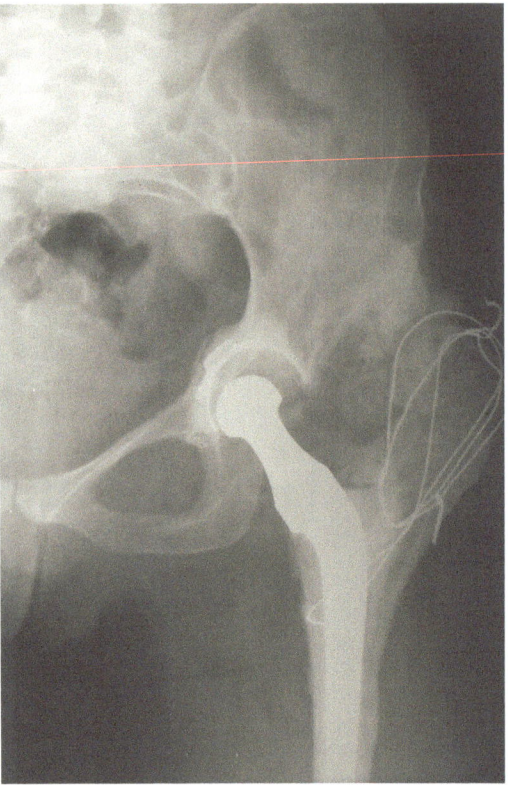

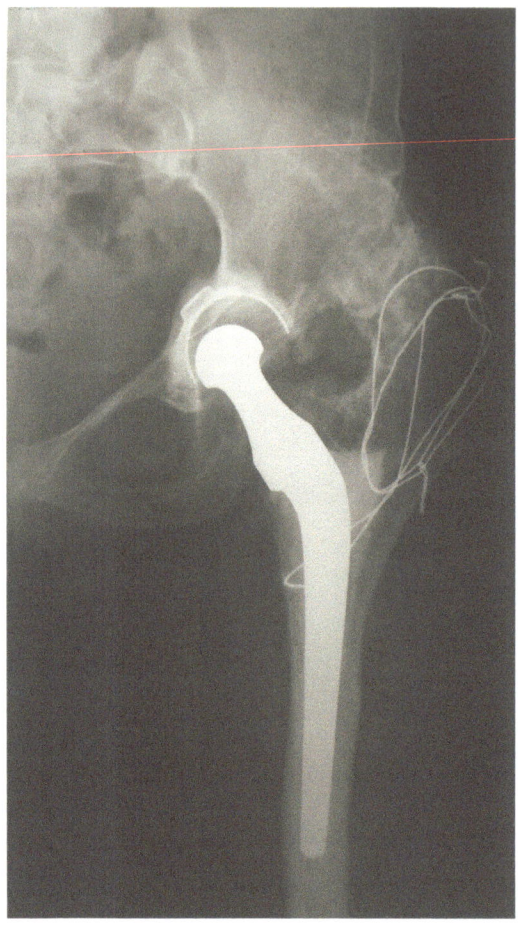

Fig 3.8 Six months postoperatively. The offset-bore acetabular component, inserted after cotyloplasty, was placed
at the level of the true acetabulum. The greater trochanter
remained in a higher position

Fig. 3.9 Twelve years after LFA

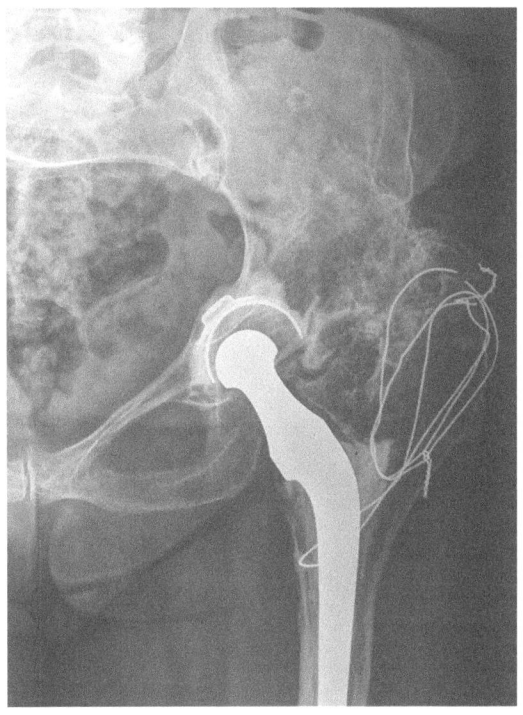

Fig. 3.10 The latest follow-up radiograph was taken 37 years after primary THR

3.3 Case 3

This female patient was born in 1955. Around the age of 25 years, she started having pain in the right hip. We first examined her in 1985, at the age of 30 years. She had moderate pain and slight limping in the right hip. The diagnosis was secondary OA because of dysplastic hip. A varus osteotomy was followed. After surgery, a slight limping remained due to 1.5 cm shortening of the right leg as a result of varus osteotomy. The fixation plate was removed 2 years later.

The patient had a normal life, without pain, for almost 20 years. Since then, she started to deteriorate, regarding pain and function, and 2 years later, when she was 52 years old, in 2007, a THR was performed 22 years after osteotomy (Figs. 3.11–3.16).

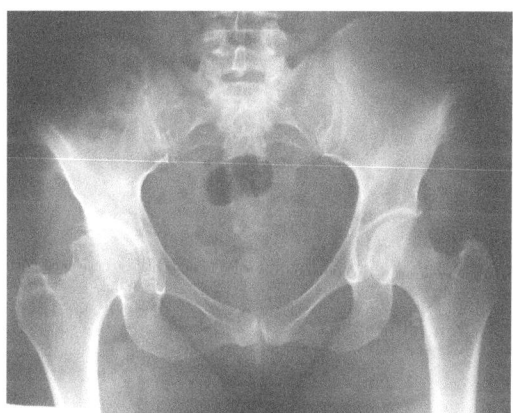

Fig. 3.11 Initial radiograph, when the patient was 30 years old, presented dysplastic right hip with early osteoarthritic changes. Varus osteotomy was followed

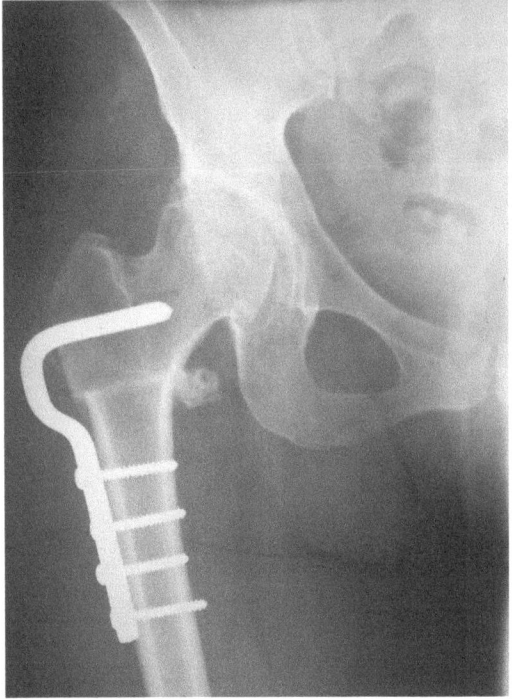

Fig. 3.12 Three months after osteotomy

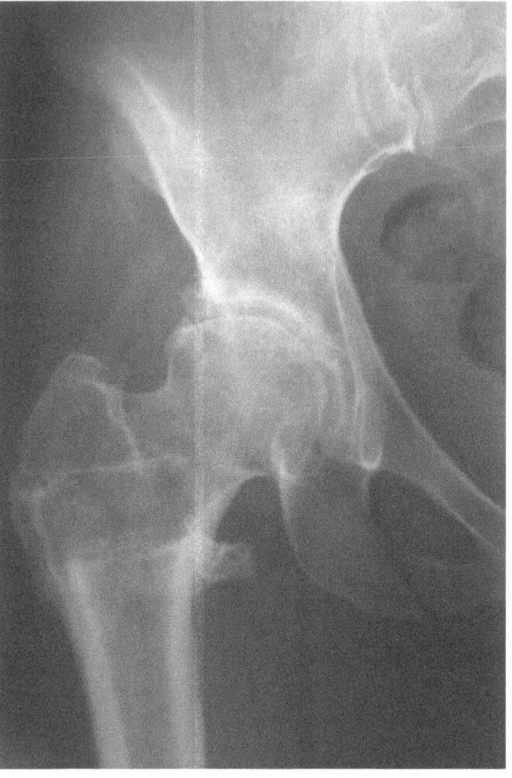

Fig. 3.14 Fifteen years after varus osteotomy. The patient remained asymptomatic and had full activities

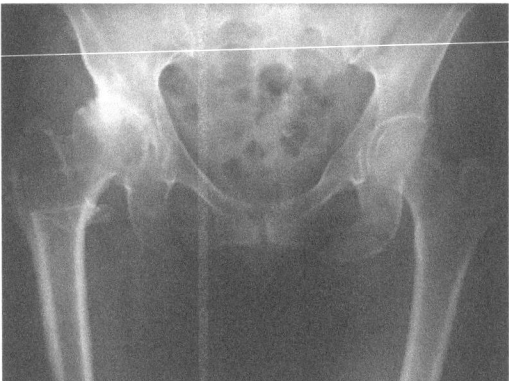

Fig. 3.15 Radiograph taken 22 years after osteotomy. The patient had started having pain and limping 2 years previously that were gradually increasing. A cementless THR was followed in 2007

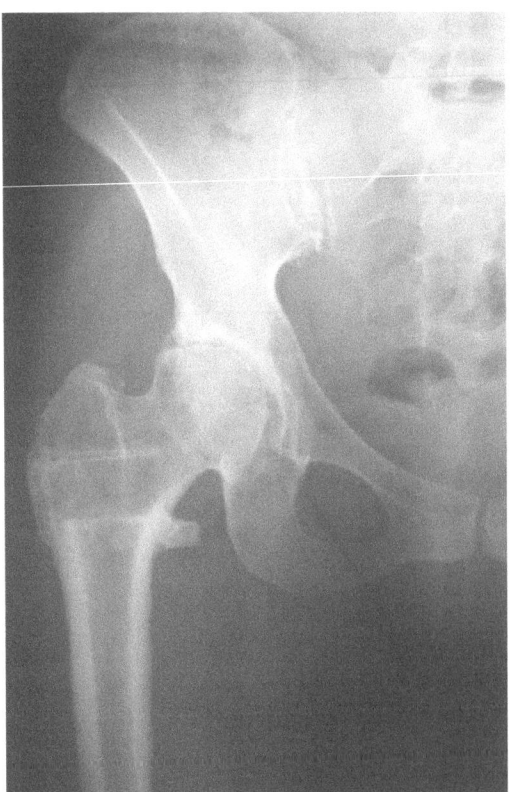

Fig. 3.13 Five years after osteotomy, the fixation plate had been removed 3 years previously

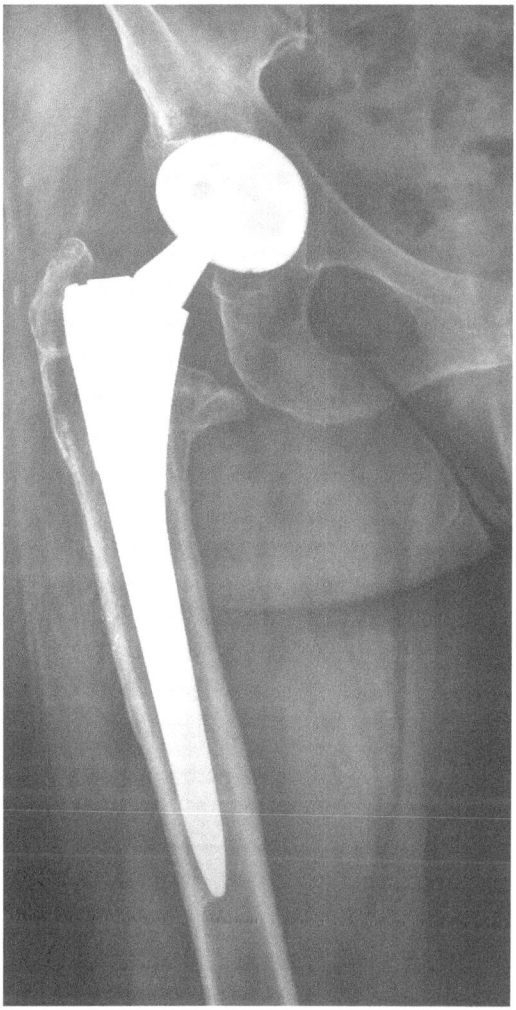

Fig. 3.16 Nine years after cementless THR. At the age of 61 years, the patient is pain-free and has full activity with a normal life

3.4   Case 4

This female patient was born in 1946. Around the age of 25 years, she started having slight pain and discomfort in the right hip. The first available radiograph, taken at the age of 29 years, revealed a dysplastic hip in the first stage of evolution of degenerative changes. The patient was referred to us 12 years later, in 1987. Pain and limping had increased. Radiograph showed that the dysplastic hip, at that time, had moderate OA. A valgus osteotomy was performed. The patient remained free of hip pain, having a slight limp for more than 15 years.

THR was needed in 2006, when the patient was 60 years old, 19 years after osteotomy. In the present, 10 years after hip replacement, she is asymptomatic and has a normal life (Figs. 3.17–3.23).

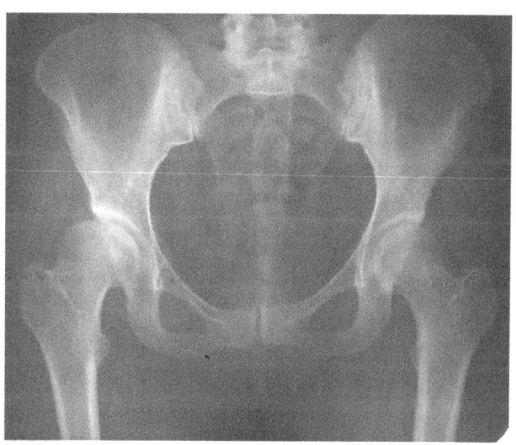

Fig. 3.17 Radiograph, when the patient was 29 years old. The right hip was dysplastic in the first stage of evolution of OA. At that time a varus osteotomy could be performed

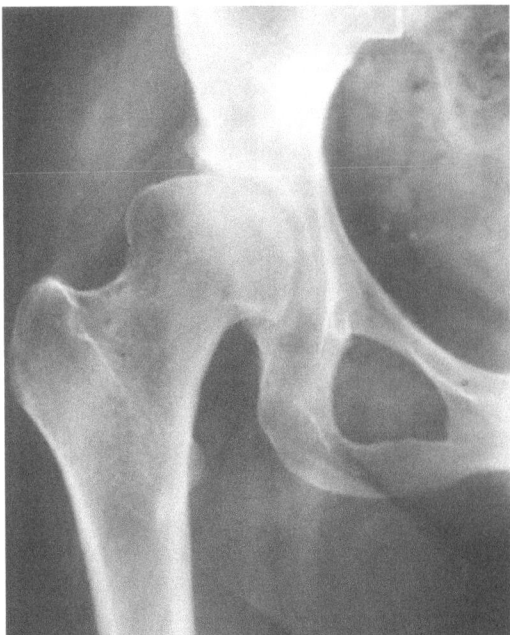

Fig. 3.18 Twelve years later, in 1987, when we first examined the patient, the dysplastic hip had progressed to the second stage of degenerative changes

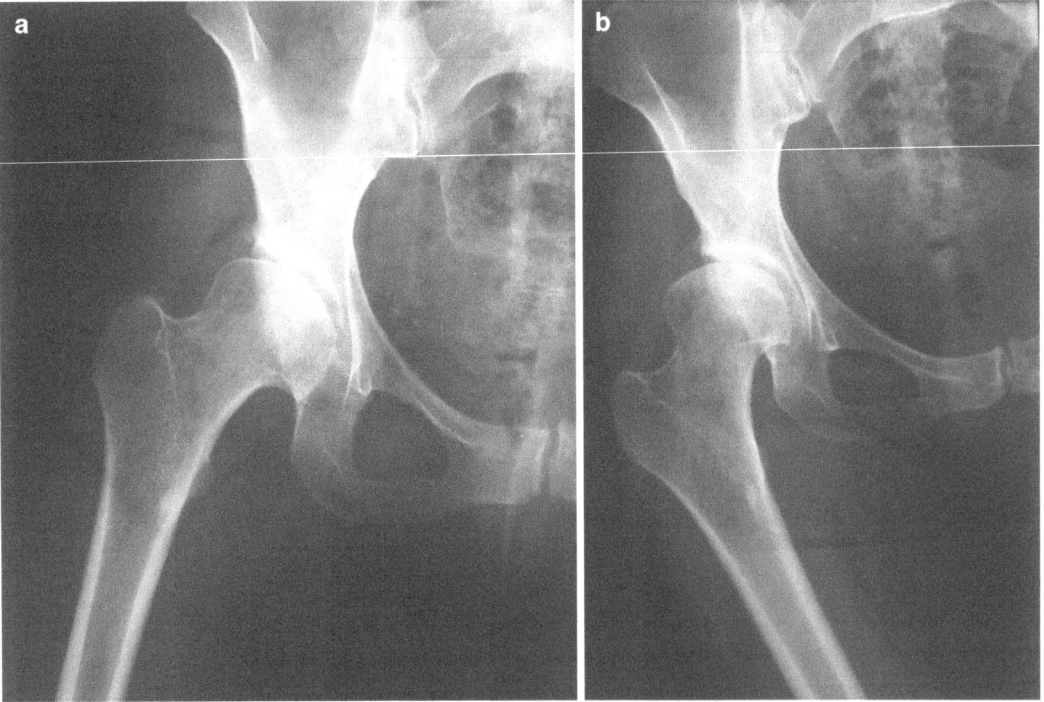

Fig. 3.19 Radiographs in (**a**) abduction and (**b**) adduction made the indication for a valgus osteotomy

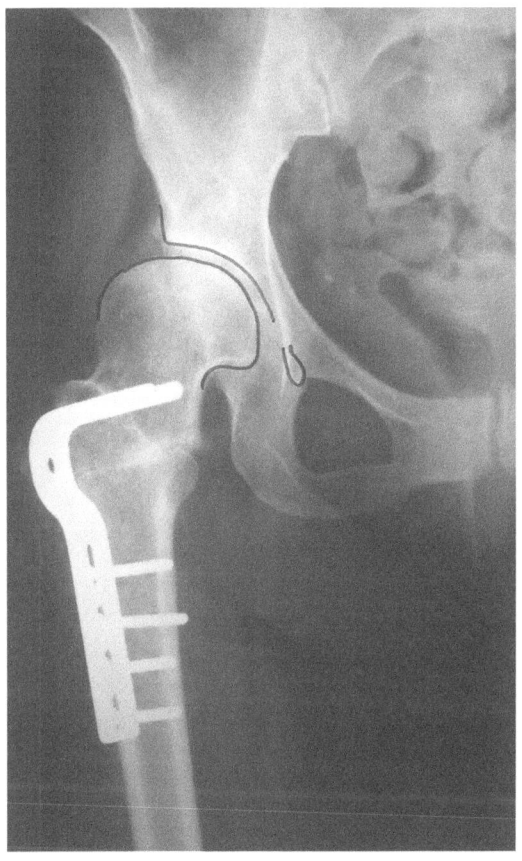

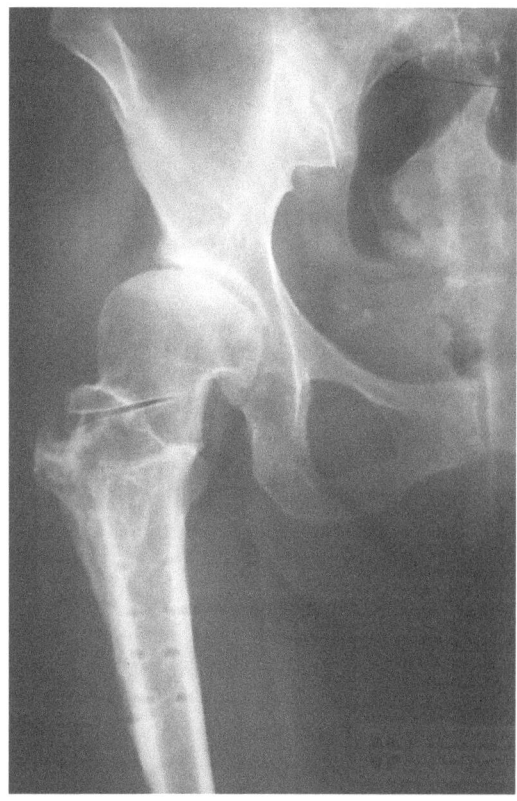

Fig. 3.21 Ten years after the valgus osteotomy, removal of implants was performed

Fig. 3.20 Postoperative radiograph

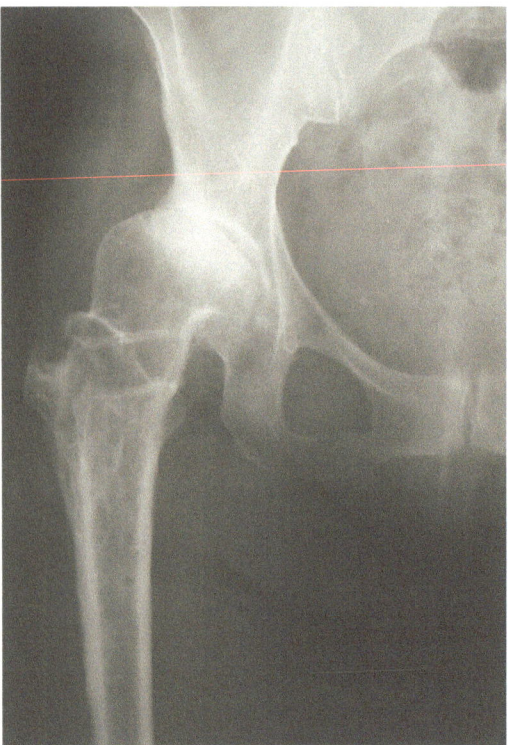

Fig. 3.22 Seventeen years after osteotomy, the patient started having increase in hip pain and limping. Two years later, in 2006, uncemented THR was performed

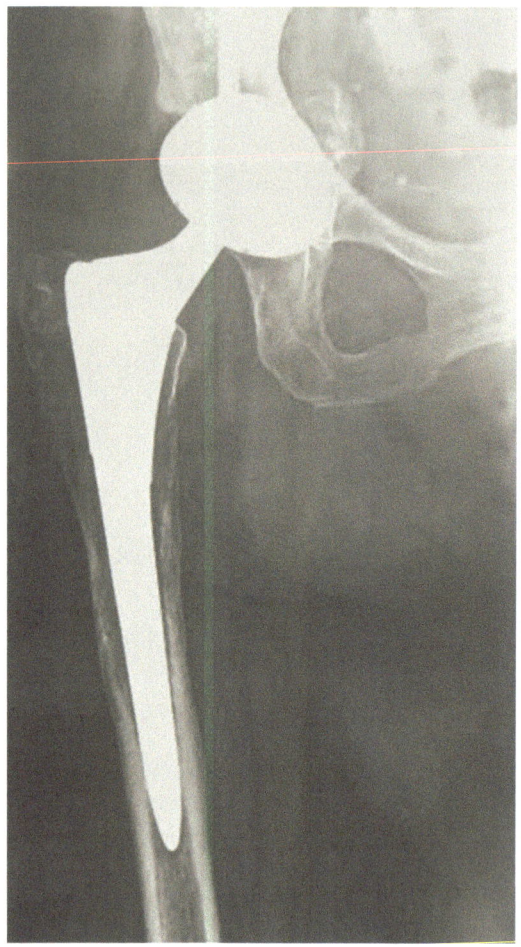

Fig. 3.23 Ten years after THR

In high dislocation, the femoral head is migrated superiorly and posteriorly in relation to the hypoplastic, triangular true acetabulum. Specifically, the acetabulum is shallow with a narrow opening and a segmental defect of the entire rim. There is also an abnormal build-up of bone posterosuperiorly and excessive anteversion. The iliac wing is also hypoplastic and anteverted. The femoral neck is short with excessive anteversion and the diaphysis is hypoplastic with excessive narrowing of the canal and thin cortices. Occasionally, there is a residual angular deformity of the proximal femur because of a previous osteotomy, which can make the reconstruction much more challenging.

We have recognised two subtypes of high dislocation in CHD, depending on the presence (C1) or the absence (C2) of a false acetabulum (Fig. 4.1). The height of the dislocation and subsequently the extent of the shortening of the femur, which is required during THR, for the reduction of components and for the avoidance of neurovascular complications, differ in the two subtypes of high dislocation.

We favour, shortening of the femur by progressive resection of bone from the femoral neck, which is a simple and uneventful technique (Fig. 4.2). We argue against leaving the greater trochanter in place and subtrochanteric femoral shortening osteotomy, because in most hips with high dislocation, the greater trochanter lies above the centre of rotation of the femoral head and its resection and advancement is important. Besides, a subtrochanteric osteotomy resembles an artificial fracture needing additional osteosynthesis that may cause undesirable complications.

In the presented cases, the extent of femoral shortening needed during the operation is estimated by subtraction of leg lengthening from the height of the dislocation and by adding or subtracting the height of the cup placement.

K. Lampropoulou-Adamidou, G. Hartofilakidis, *Total Hip Replacement*,
DOI 10.1007/978-3-319-53360-5_4

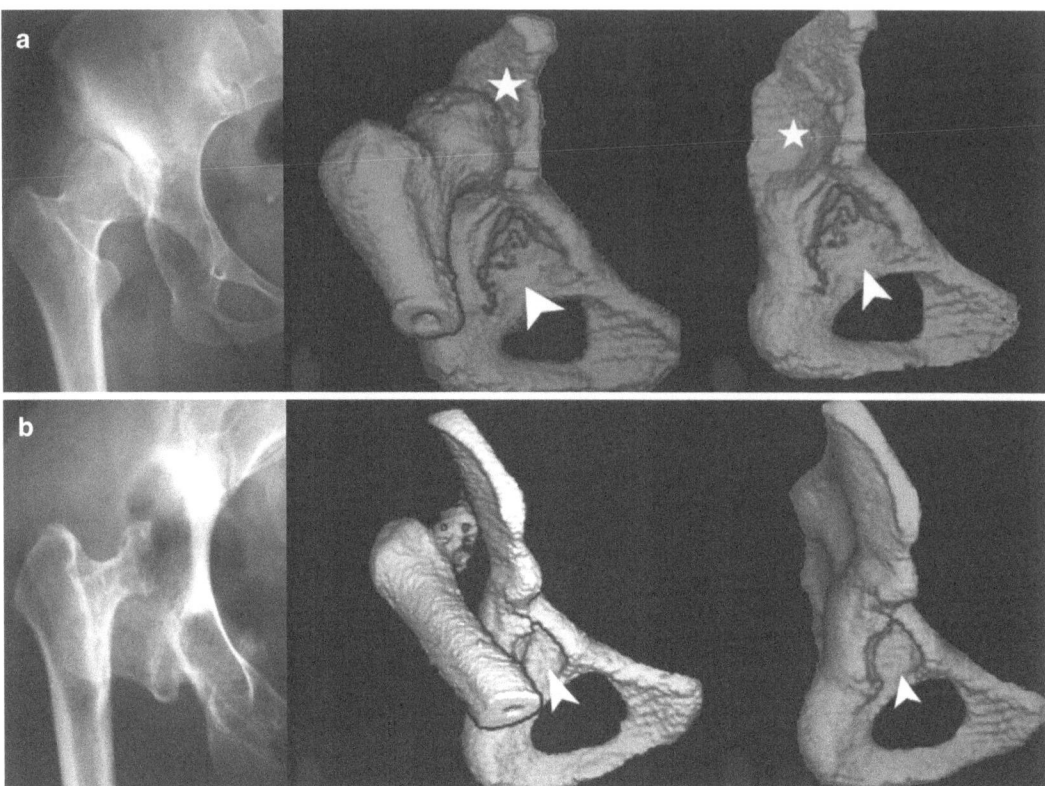

Fig 4.1 The radiological appearance and the 3D CT scan, with and without the femoral head, in the two subtypes of high dislocation. (**a**) C1 subtype high dislocation in which the false acetabulum is denoted by a *star* and the true acetabulum by an *arrow* and (**b**) C2 subtype high dislocation with no false acetabulum; the femoral head is free-floating within the gluteal muscles. An *arrow* marks the true acetabulum

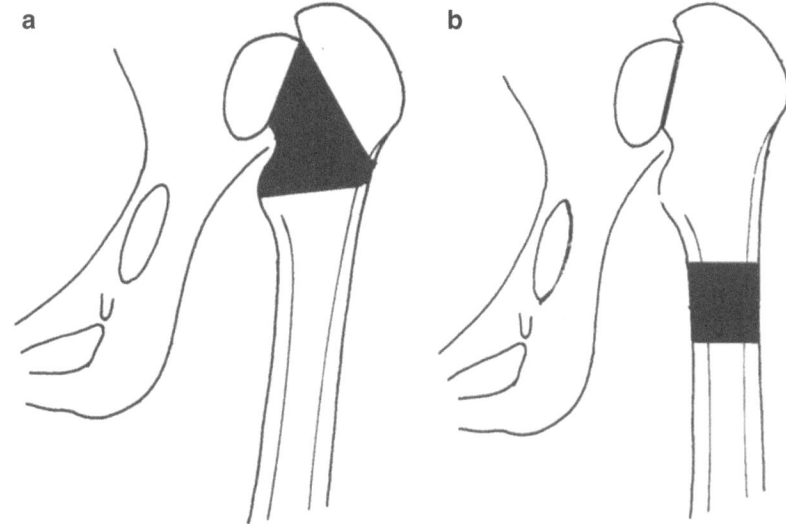

Fig 4.2 Drawings of the two main alternative methods of femoral shortening: (**a**) at the level of the femoral neck and (**b**) distal shortening at the level of the femoral shaft

4.1   Case 1

This female patient was born in 1958 with complete dislocation of both hips. At the age of 2 years, she was treated by her physician with closed reduction and prolonged immobilisation in plaster. Ever since then, she had severe limping. The first available radiograph, taken when she was 12 years old, showed that both hips remained completely dislocated.

We first examined her, in 1987, when she was 29 years old. She had C2 subtype high dislocation bilaterally. Her main complaint was the severe limping and the persistent low-back pain, symptoms that, in consultation with us, despite her young age, led to the decision for THRs. She had bilateral LFAs within 3 months. Her life changed radically. She had a normal life with only slight limping in the right hip. At the age of 37 years, she married and she gave birth to a healthy boy.

Twenty-seven years postoperatively, in 2014, she sustained dislocation of the right hip, treated with revision of both components. At the last follow-up examination, 29 years after primary THR of the left hip and 2 years after revision of the right hip, she remained without hip pain and had full activity level with only a slight limp (Figs. 4.3–4.8).

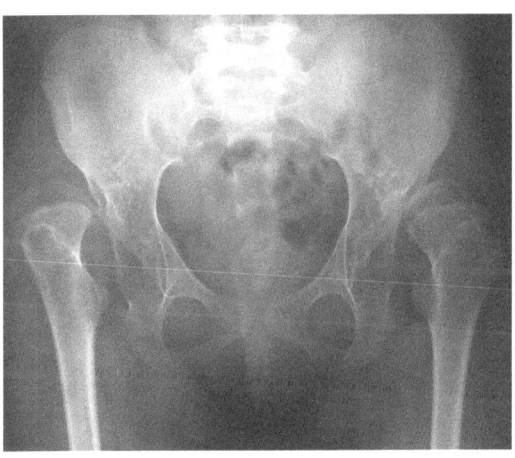

Fig. 4.3 Radiograph, when the patient was 12 years old

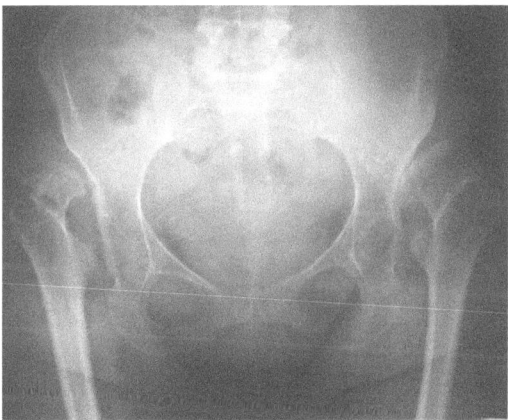

Fig. 4.4 Preoperative radiograph taken in 1987, when she was 29 years old. She had C2 subtype high dislocation bilaterally. The height of the dislocation was 6 cm in both hips

Fig. 4.5 Early
postoperative
radiographs. Four
centimetre shortening in
both femurs had been
required

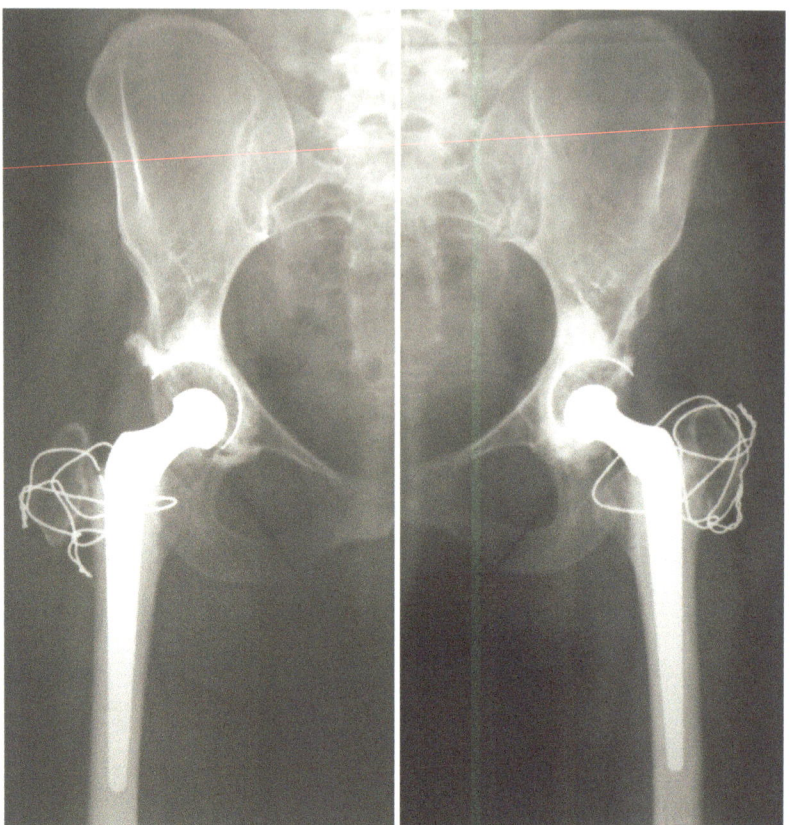

Fig. 4.6 Fifteen years postoperatively

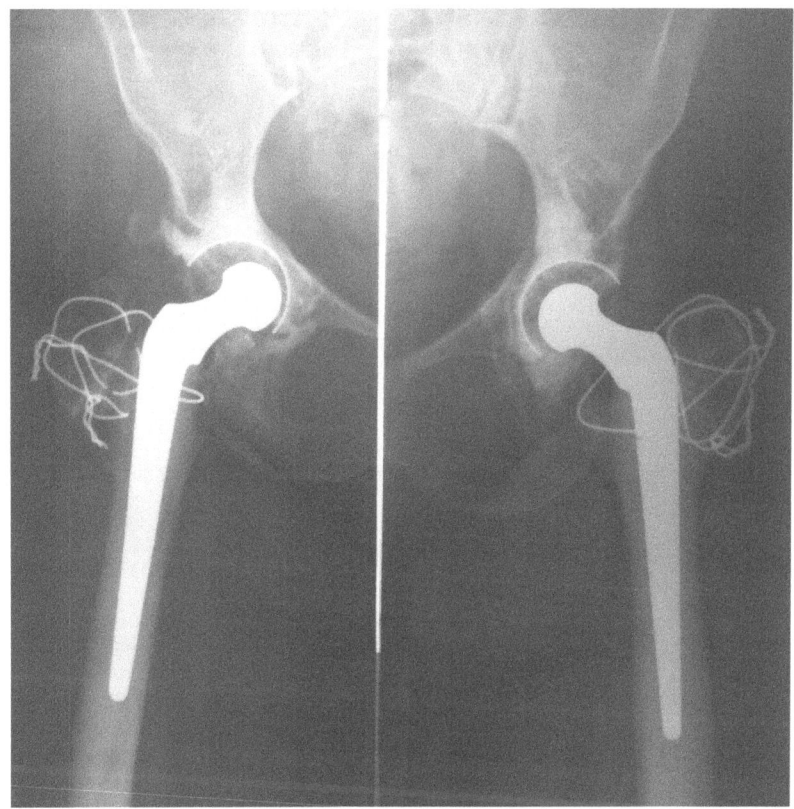

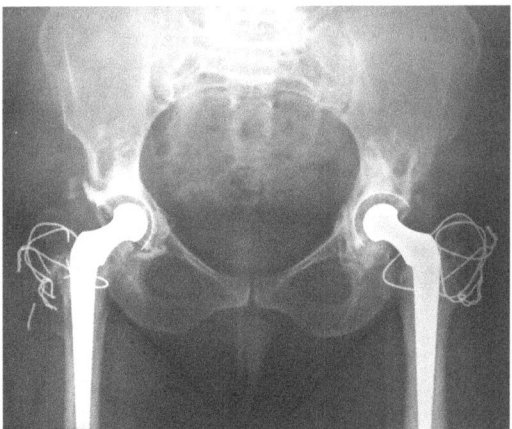

Fig. 4.7 Radiograph 26 years postoperatively, there is acetabular wear in both hips, especially in the right. One year later, she sustained dislocation of the right hip, treated with revision of both components

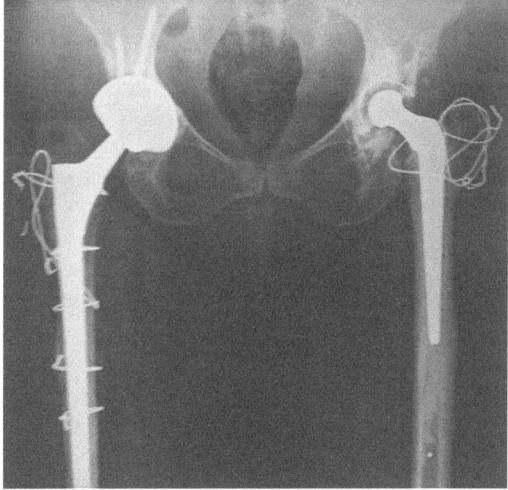

Fig. 4.8 The last follow-up radiograph taken 2 years after revision of the right hip and 29 years after primary THR of the left. Note that the acetabular wear of the left hip has increased. More frequent follow-up of the patient was recommended

4.2   Case 2

This female patient was born in 1942 with bilateral CHD. She remained without treatment and she was limping since infancy. We first examined her, when she was 47 years old, in 1989. She had severe limping and pain. The diagnosis was bilateral C2 subtype high dislocation. She had LFA in both hips within 1 month. The offset-bore acetabular component, inserted after cotyloplasty, and the Harris CDH stem were used in both hips. She gained painless hips, while a slight limping remained.

The 20-year follow-up radiograph revealed initiation of acetabular wear and linear osteolysis around the right cup that progressed during the following years. As a result, the cup started to migrate and the patient began to have hip pain and increase in limping. Revision of acetabular component of the right hip was followed. At the 27th-year follow-up, the patient is 74 years old, free of hip pain and walks with a use of cane in the left hand (Figs. 4.9–4.14).

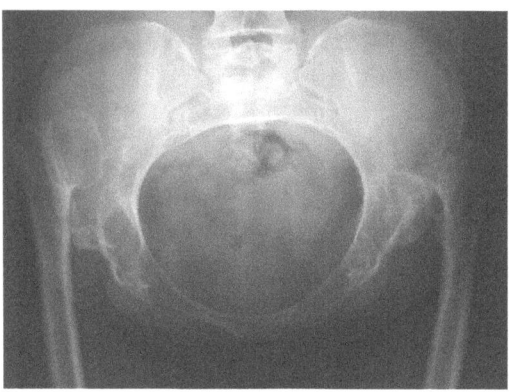

Fig. 4.9 Preoperative radiograph. The height of the dislocation was 8 cm in the left and 7 cm in the right hip

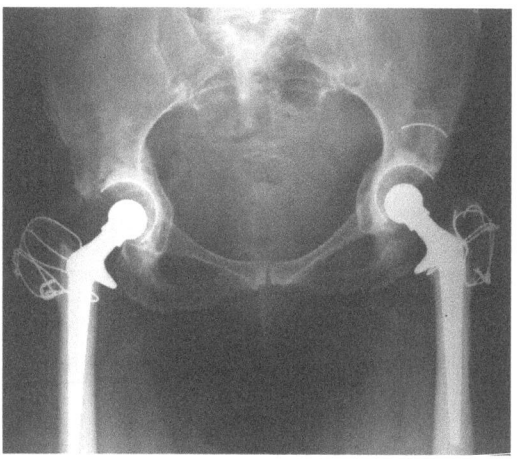

Fig. 4.11 Ten years after surgery

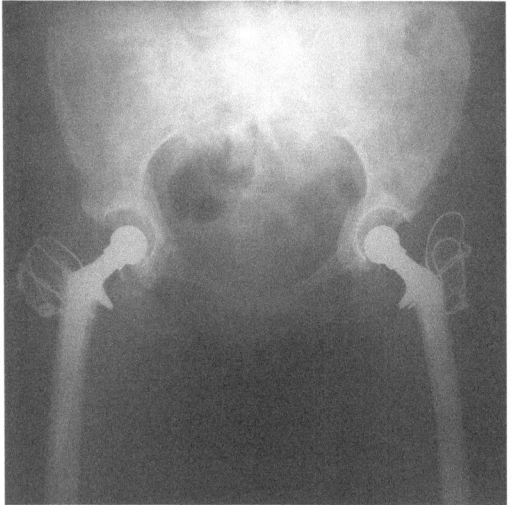

Fig. 4.10 Early postoperative radiographs. The left femur was shortened 3 cm and the right 2 cm

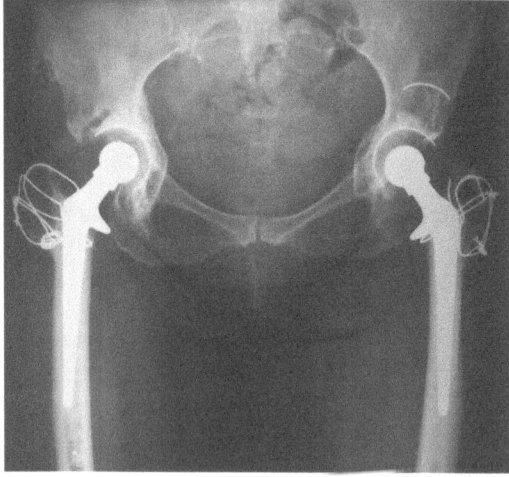

Fig. 4.12 Twenty years after surgery, when the acetabular wear and linear osteolysis around the right acetabular component were noted

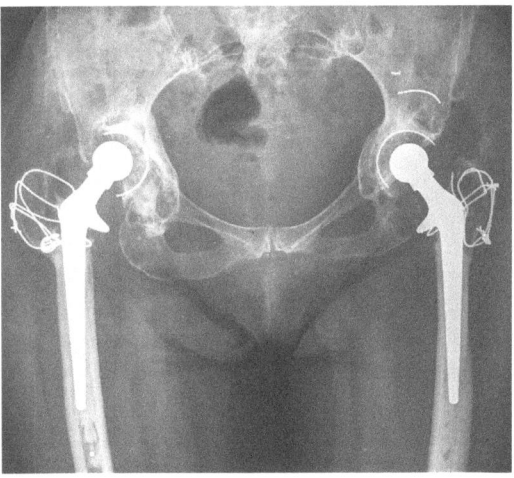

Fig. 4.13 Radiograph taken 26 years after primary THRs. The right cup had migrated. The patient had increase in limping and pain. The left hip had wear of the cup without osteolysis and was asymptomatic. Revision of the right hip was followed in another institution

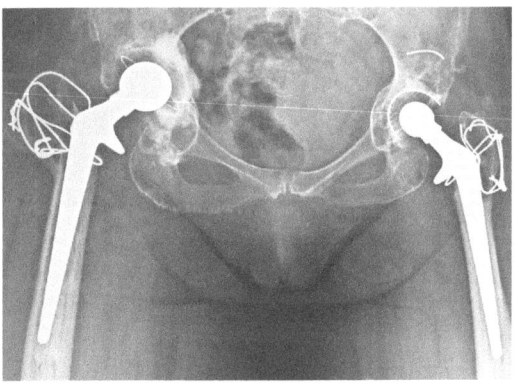

Fig. 4.14 One year after revision of the right acetabular component and 27 years after left primary THR

4.3   Case 3

This female patient was born in 1958 with complete dislocation of both hips. She had no treatment in infancy. She was referred to us in 1989, at the age of 31 years. She had bilateral high dislocation of the C2 subtype. Her main compliant was the heavy limping. The decision for surgery was made after repeated consultations, considering mainly the psychological impact. Two years later, a hybrid THR was performed in both hips within 40 days.

Fourteen years after surgery, revision of both polyethylene liners was decided because of progressive wear, in order to avoid development of osteolysis, despite the fact that the patient was asymptomatic. Twenty-four years after primary surgery, in 2015, right stem and polyethylene revision was also performed, because of femoral component's aseptic loosening. At the latest follow-up evaluation, 25 years after primary THRs, the patient was free of symptoms and had normal activities (Figs. 4.15–4.20).

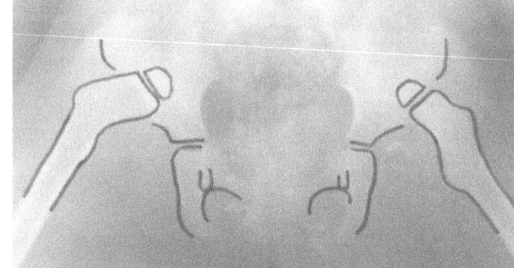

Fig. 4.15 Radiograph, when the patient was 2 years old

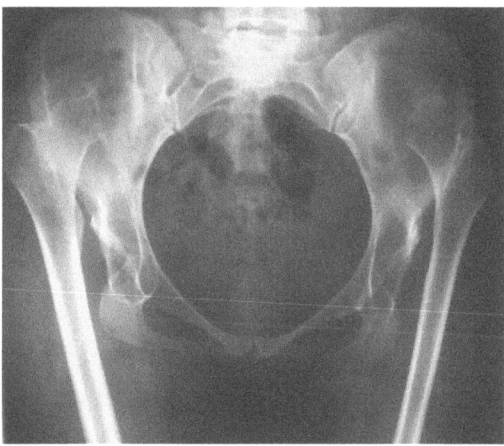

Fig. 4.16 Preoperative radiograph in 1991, at the age of 33 years. The height of the dislocation was 9 cm in both hips

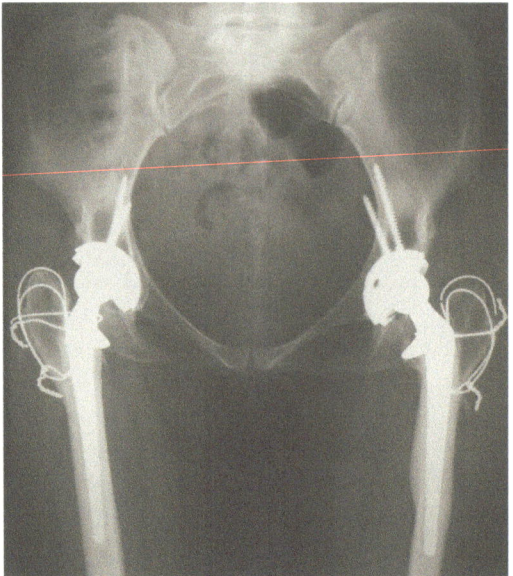

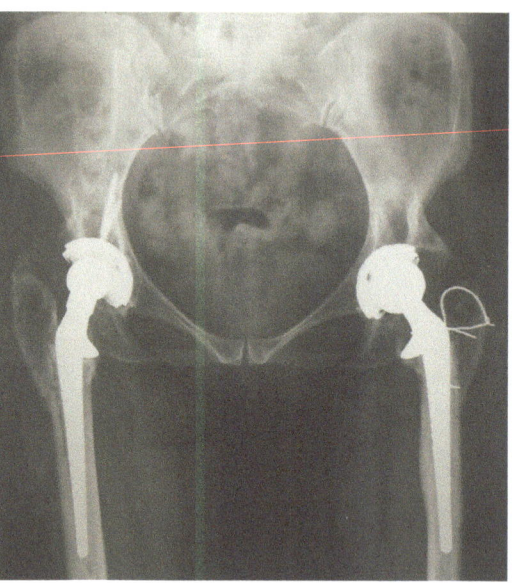

Fig. 4.17 Ten years after hybrid THRs. Six and 7 cm shortening of the femur of the left and right hip, respectively, was needed in order to reduce the hips and obtain normal centre of rotation

Fig. 4.19 Radiograph taken in 2015, 24 years after primary replacements and 10 years after exchange of polyethylene liners. Revision of the right femoral component and a new exchange of the polyethylene were considered necessary

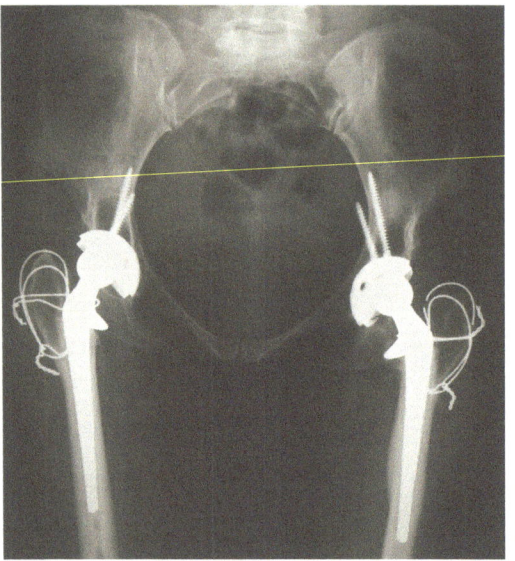

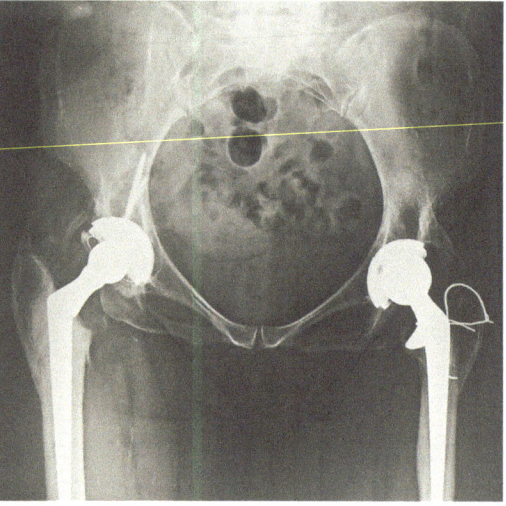

Fig. 4.18 Fourteen years postoperatively. Note the presence of significant wear of both polyethylene liners without osteolysis. One-stage bilateral exchange of liners was performed. In addition in the left hip, acetabular screws were removed, and the femoral head was replaced with a larger one because the hip intraoperatively was considered unstable

Fig. 4.20 Radiograph 1 year after femoral and polyethylene liner revision of the right hip and 25 years after primary THRs. Both acetabular shells and the left stem are in place from the primary THRs

4.4   Case 4

This female patient was born in 1940 with bilateral CHD. She had no treatment in infancy and she was limping since then. She was referred to us, at the age of 40 years, in 1980, with low dislocation of the right hip and high dislocation of the left. She was treated with LFA of the right hip in 1980, at the age of 40 years, and 5 years later of the left hip. At the present, she is 76 years old, and she remains asymptomatic, without pain and limping, 36 and 31 years after THR, respectively (Figs. 4.21–4.23).

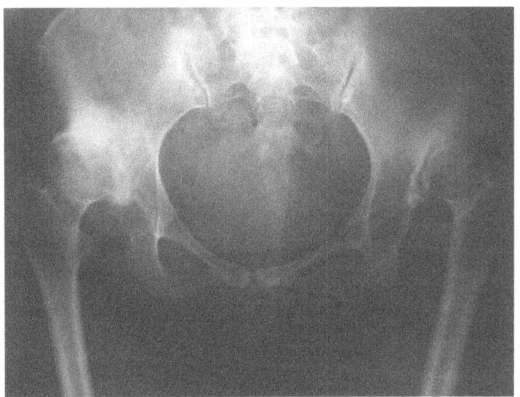

Fig. 4.21 Preoperative radiograph presented low dislocation of the right hip and C1 subtype high dislocation of the left hip, which had 4 cm dislocation height

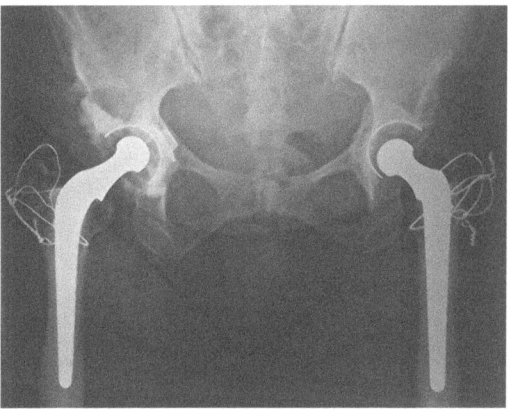

Fig 4.23 The latest available follow-up radiograph, 30 and 25 years, after THR of the right and left hip, respectively

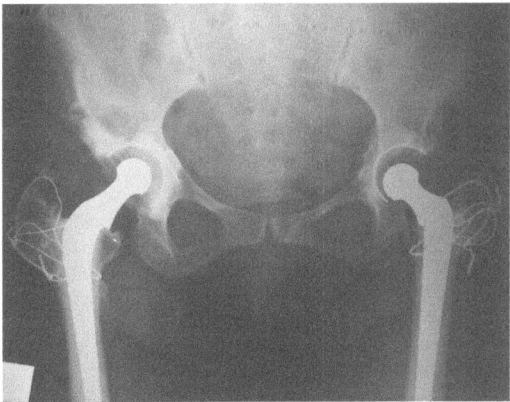

Fig. 4.22 Nine and 4 years after LFA of the right and left hip, respectively. Shortening of the hips was not required. The cotyloplasty technique was used in both hips

4.5   Case 5

This female patient was born in 1938 with congenital disease of the left hip. She had no treatment in infancy. She was limping since then, and around the age of 30 years, she began having pain in the left hip. The deterioration was slow and the patient referred to us when she was 52 years old. She had high dislocation of the C1 subtype. THR was per-

formed in 1990 using the offset-bore cup, inserted after cotyloplasty, and Charnley CDH stem.

At the 20-year follow-up examination, polyethylene wear and linear osteolysis around the acetabular component were noticed. The following years, the cup started to migrate proximally. Symptoms, pain and limping, appeared suddenly in 2016, 26 years postoperatively. The patient has been planned for revision (Figs. 4.24–4.29).

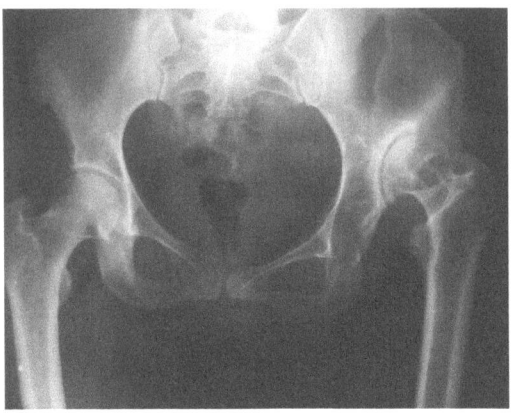

Fig. 4.24 Preoperative radiograph. The height of the dislocation was 5 cm

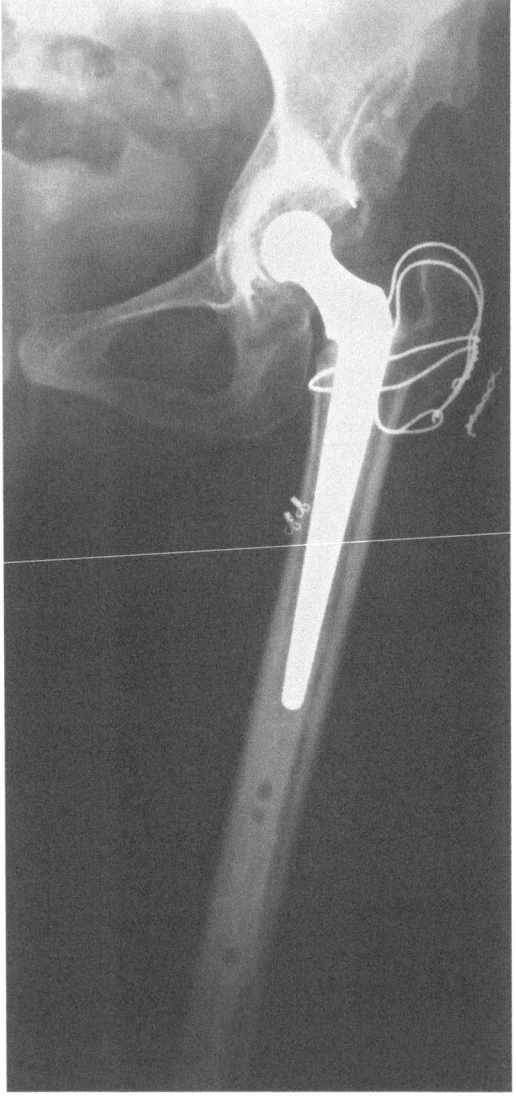

Fig. 4.25 Three years postoperatively. The femur was shortened 1 cm. During insertion of the cement with a gun, the cement plug moved distally and the cement escaped several centimetres. As a result the cement mantle became insufficient

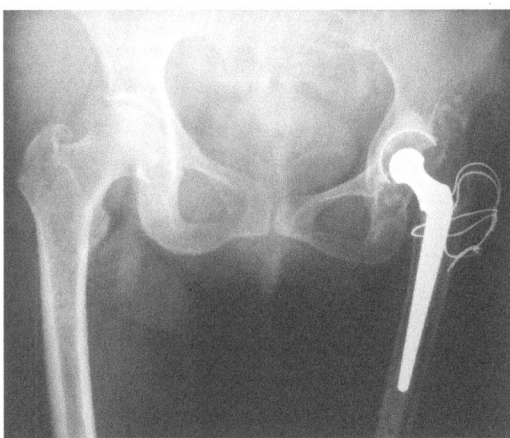

Fig. 4.26 The 18th postoperative year, although there is osteolysis around the stem and cement is only visible in Gruen zone 4, there was no stem migration nor polyethylene wear

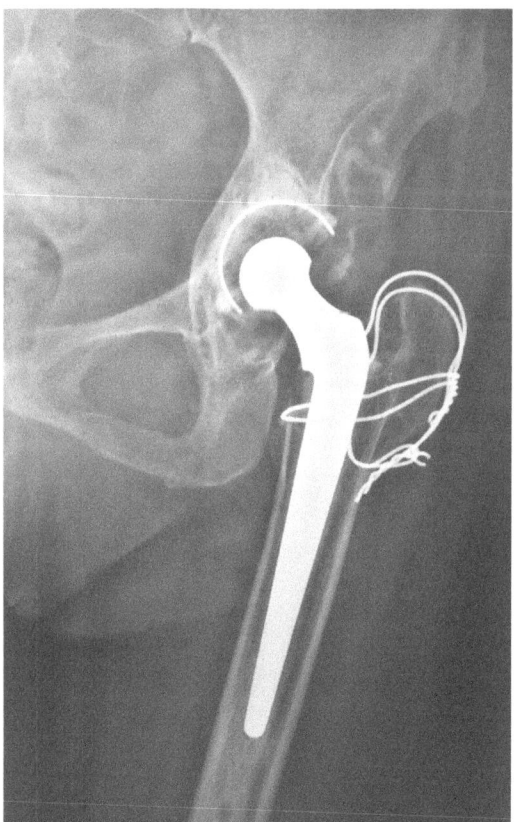

Fig. 4.27 Twenty years postoperatively, the first evidence of cup wear was present

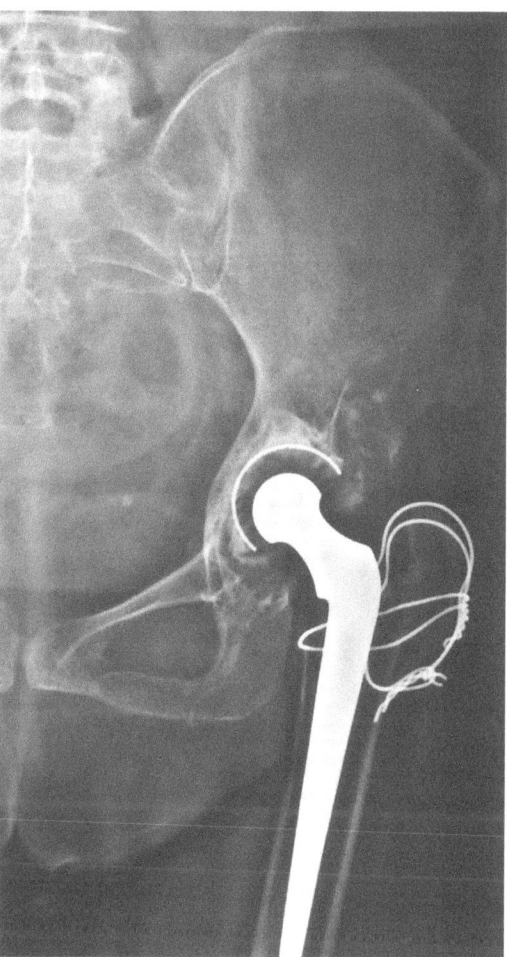

Fig. 4.28 Radiograph of the 24th postoperative year. The cup had slightly migrated

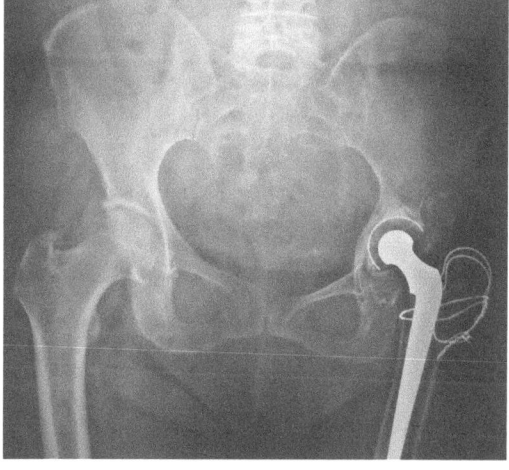

Fig. 4.29 The latest follow-up radiograph was taken 26 years after primary surgery. Migration of the cup had increased and the patient became symptomatic, at the age of 78 years. She is scheduled for revision

4.6   Case 6

This female patient was born in 1928 with complete dislocation of the left hip. At the age of 35 years, in 1963, she underwent by her physician

a Schanz osteotomy. We performed a THR, when she was 62 years old, in 1990. At the last contact with the patient via phone, when she was 85 years old, she reported activity compatible to her age without hip pain (Figs. 4.30–4.32).

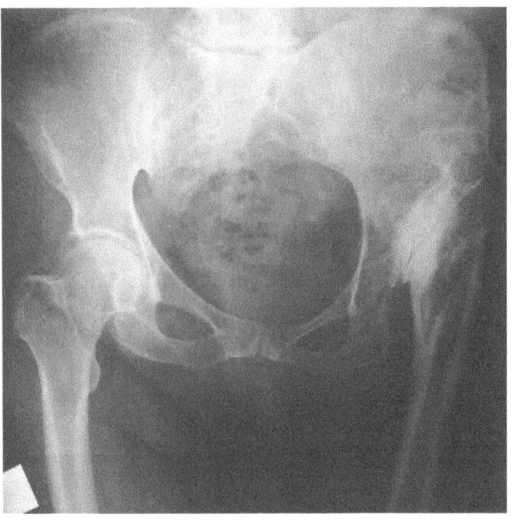

Fig. 4.30 Radiograph taken before LFA in 1990. The height of the dislocation was 9 cm

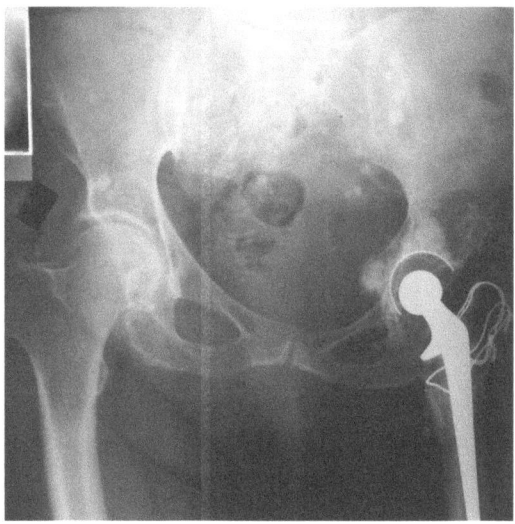

Fig. 4.32 The latest available follow-up radiograph, 20 years postoperatively

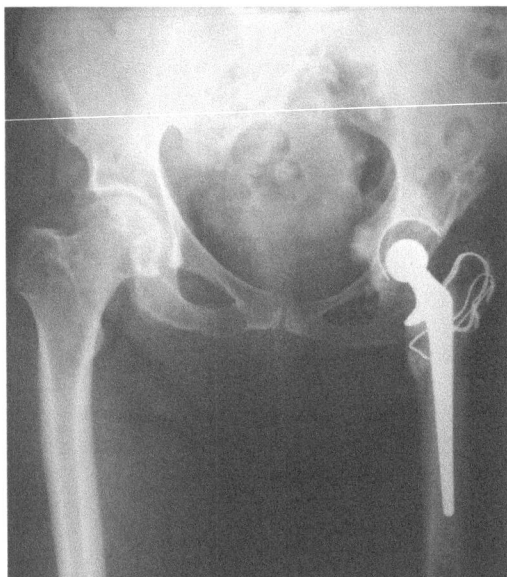

Fig. 4.31 Two years postoperatively. The offset-bore acetabulum inserted with cotyloplasty and the Harris CDH stem were used. The femur was shortened 4 cm

4.7   Case 7

This female patient was born in 1951 with bilateral CHD. She had no treatment in infancy. She had severe limping since then and hip pain started around the age of 35. We examined her at the age of 42 years. She had C1 subtype high dislocation of the right hip and low dislocation of the left. Hybrid THR of both hips was performed within 1 month, in 1993. At the last follow-up examination, 23 years postoperatively, she had no hip pain and retained normal activity. A slight limp remained on the left leg (Figs. 4.33–4.36).

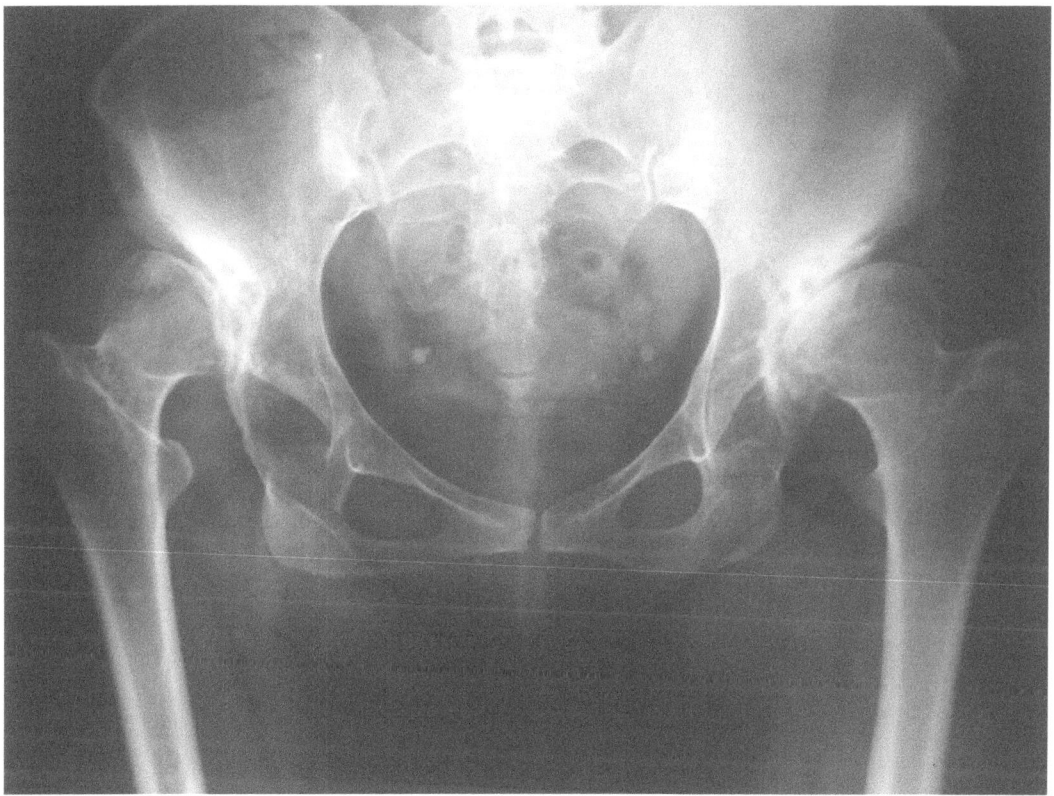

Fig. 4.33 Preoperative radiograph. The right hip was classified as having C1 subtype high dislocation of 4 cm height and the left as having low dislocation

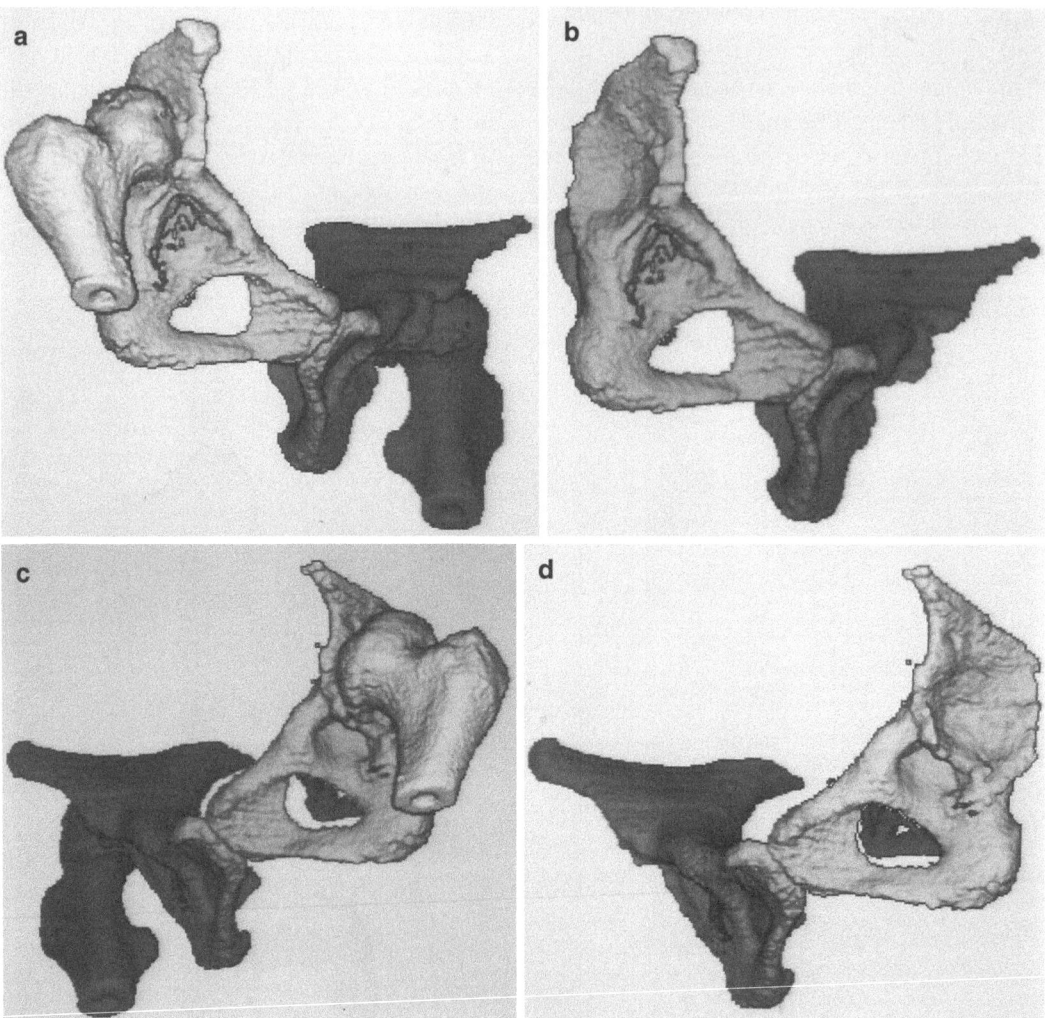

Fig. 4.34 Three-dimensional CT scans of the right and the left hip (**a**, **c**) with and (**b**, **d**) without the femoral head

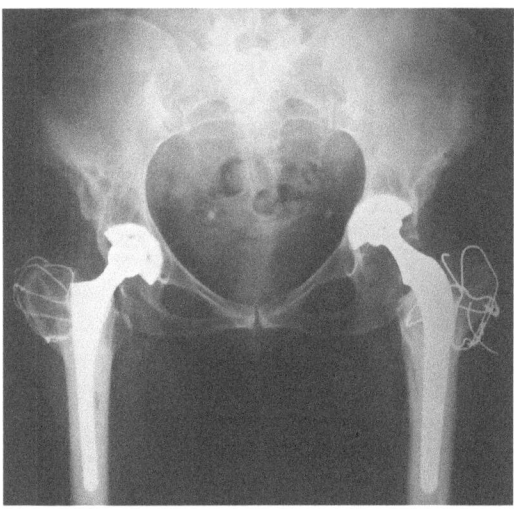

Fig. 4.35 Ten years postoperatively. The needed shortening of the right femur was 3 cm

4.8   Case 8

This female patient was born in 1954 with complete dislocation of the right hip. She received no treatment in infancy. She was limping since then, while pain in both hips started around the age of 30 years. She had secondary OA of the right hip because of C1 subtype high dislocation and of the left hip because of dysplasia. Rapid worsening of symptoms occurred in the left hip, and the patient referred to us at the age of 40 years, in 1994. Hybrid THR of the left and the right hip was performed within 3 months. The latest follow-up evaluation was performed 22 years after primary replacements. The patient was free of hip pain without limping and had a normal activity level (Figs. 4.37–4.40).

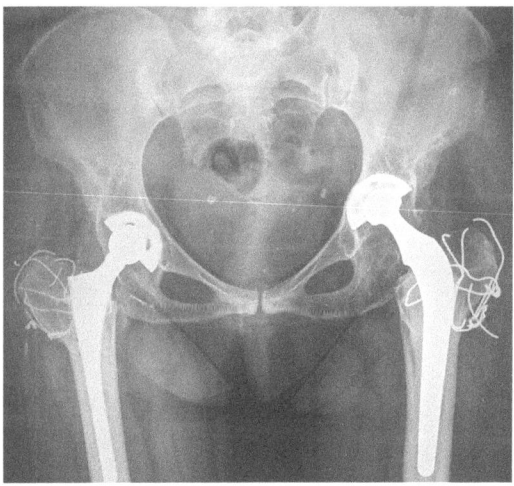

Fig. 4.36 The last follow-up radiograph taken 23 years postoperatively

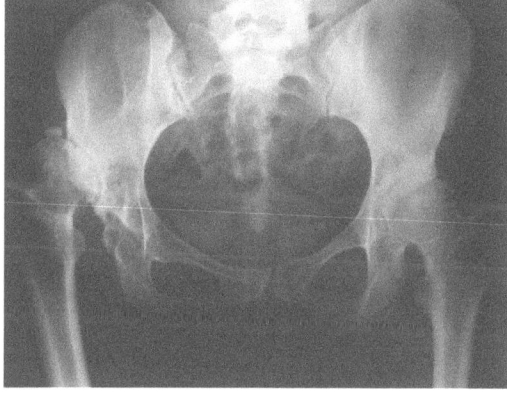

Fig. 4.37 Radiograph taken in 1989 when the patient was 35 years old. She had mild pain in both hips. The right hip was classified as having C1 subtype high dislocation and the left hip as having dysplasia with mild secondary OA. The height of the dislocation of the right hip was 2 cm

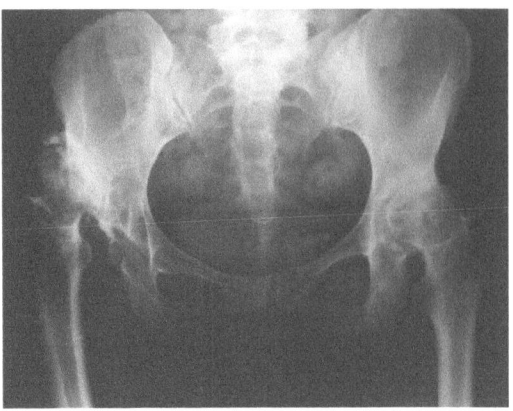

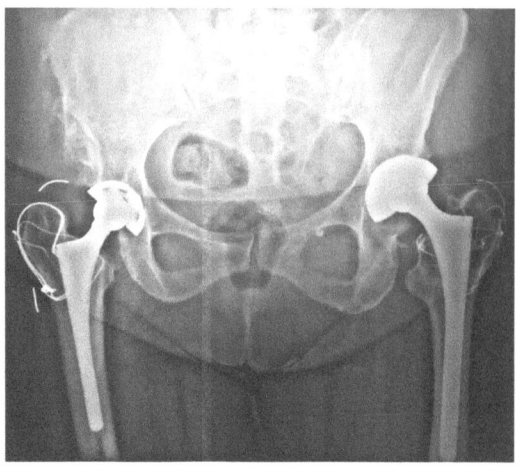

Fig. 4.38 Radiograph, taken 5 years later. The deterioration of both hips was remarkable. THR of both hips within 3 months was followed

Fig. 4.40 The latest follow-up radiograph taken 22 years after primary replacements

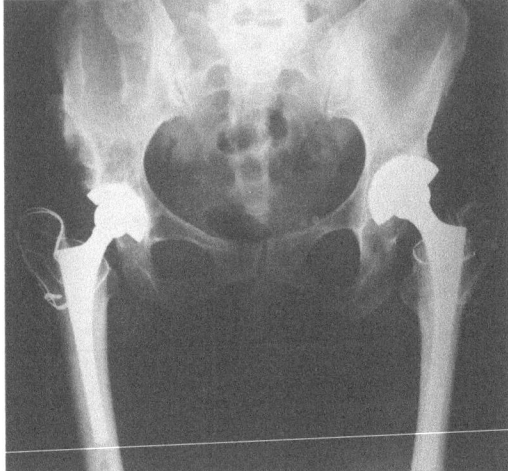

Fig. 4.39 Radiograph taken at the third-year follow-up examination. Shortening of the right femur was not needed

4.9 Case 9

This female patient was born in 1938 with bilateral CHD. She had no treatment in infancy. She was limping on the left side. Pain first started in the right hip around the age of 20 years. We first examined her when she was 54 years old in 1992. She had a C2 subtype high dislocation of the left hip and low dislocation with severe secondary OA of the right hip. Hybrid THR was performed in the right side followed after 9 months by the same procedure in the left. Three months after the latter procedure, the left hip was dislocated, because the cup had been placed in extreme vertical position. This complication was faced with acetabular component revision.

For the next 23 years until the last follow-up examination, the patient remained without hip pain. In the last 5 years, she experienced severe neurological symptoms from both lower extremities because of lumbar spinal stenosis (Figs. 4.41–4.46).

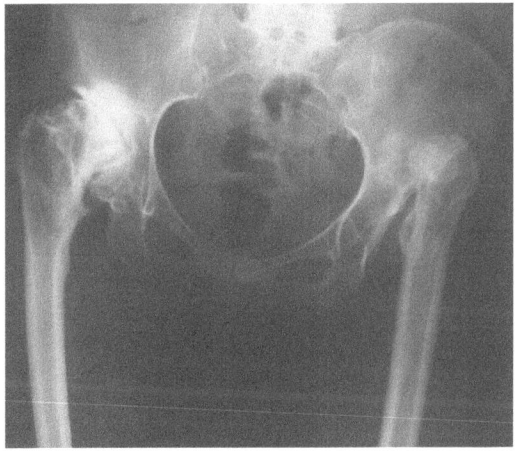

Fig. 4.41 Preoperative radiograph. There was a C2 subtype high dislocation of the left hip and low dislocation of the right. The height of the dislocation of the left hip was 6 cm

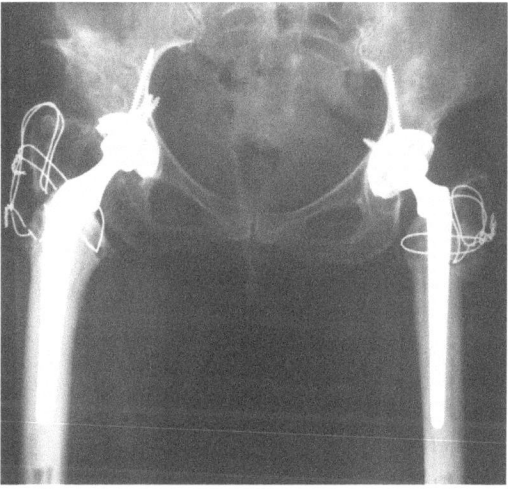

Fig. 4.43 Fourteen months after right primary THR and 2 months after left cup revision

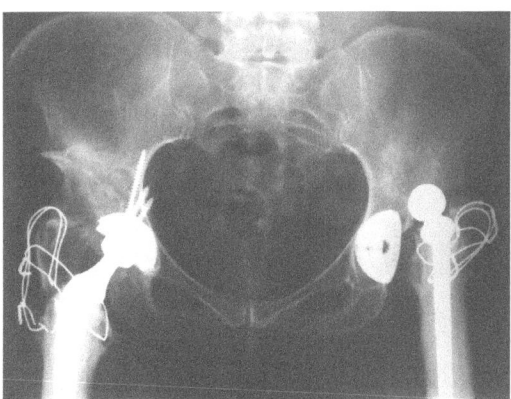

Fig. 4.42 Intraoperative shortening of the left femur had not been required. The left hip was dislocated 3 months postoperatively, and acetabular component revision was followed

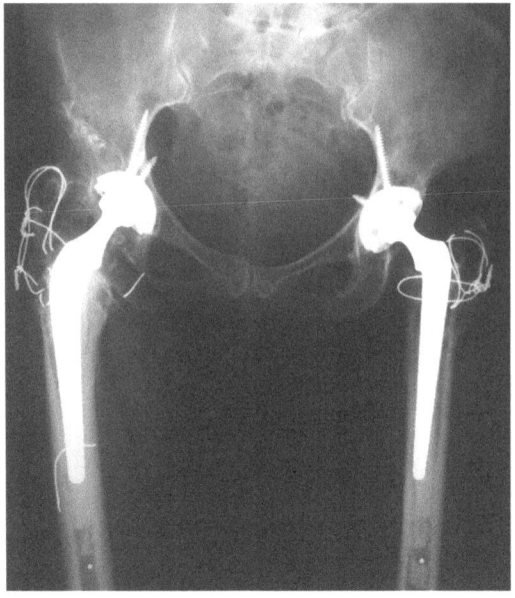

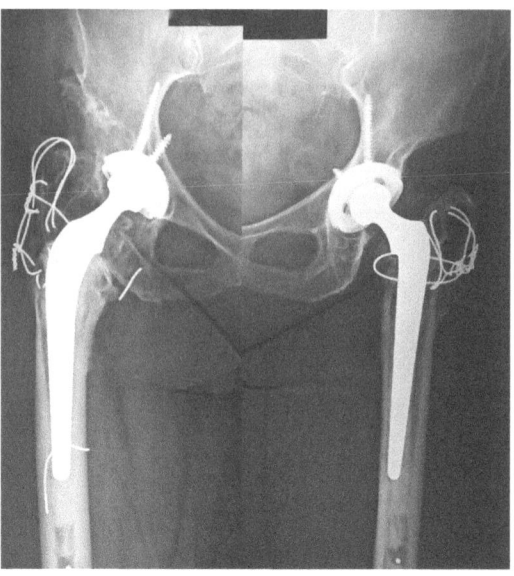

Fig. 4.45 Nineteen years postoperatively. The left stem was considered as possibly loose

Fig. 4.44 Radiograph taken at the 16th-year follow-up examination

Fig. 4.46 The last follow-up radiograph, 23 years postoperatively. Loosening of the left stem progressed (probably loose) without migration. The patient remains without hip symptoms

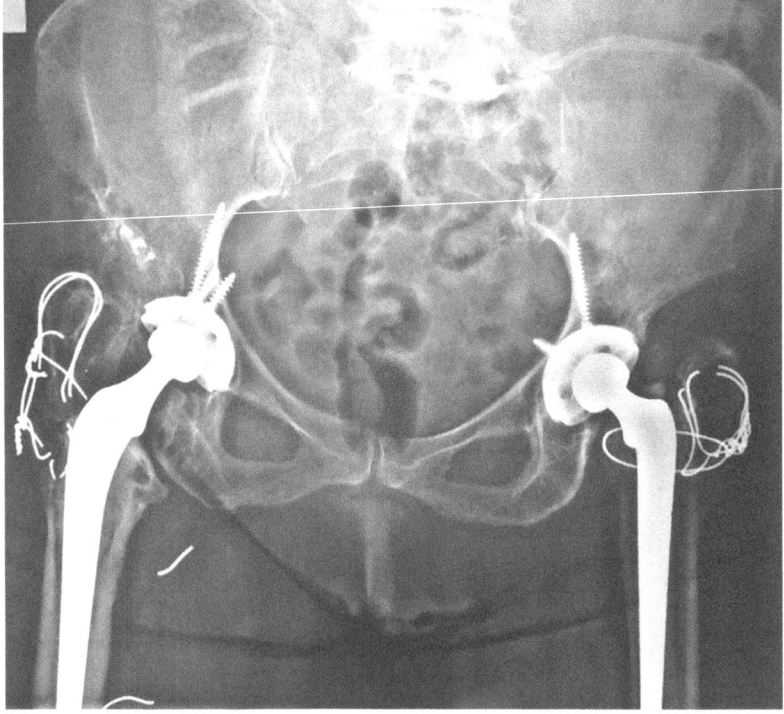

4.10   Case 10

This female patient was born in 1957 with complete dislocation of the left hip. She had no treatment in infancy. Hip pain started around the age of 20 years. We performed a cementless THR for C1 subtype high dislocation, when the patient was 34 years old in 1991.

Thirteen years postoperatively, an extensive polyethylene wear was observed and a polyethylene liner exchange was performed, although the patient was asymptomatic.

Twenty-five years from primary replacement, the patient was 59 years old, she walked without hip pain or limping, and she lived a normal life (Figs. 4.47–4.50).

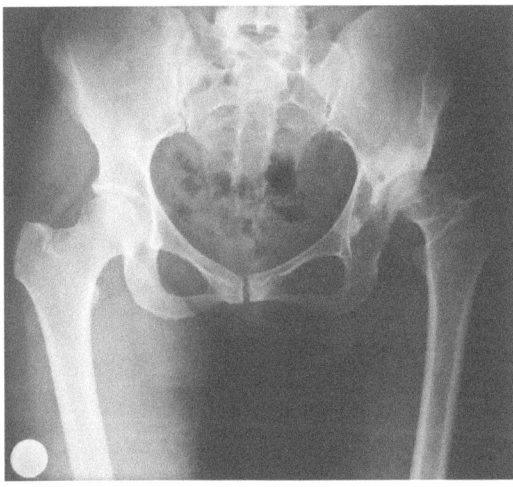

Fig. 4.47 Preoperative radiograph. There is a C1 subtype high dislocation of the left hip with 3 cm height

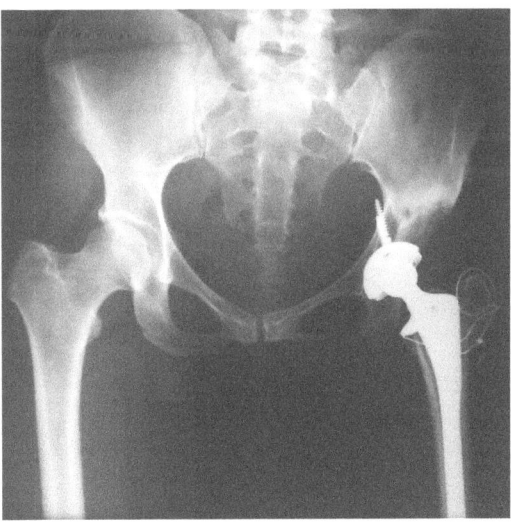

Fig. 4.48 Three months after cementless THR. One centimetre of femoral shortening was needed

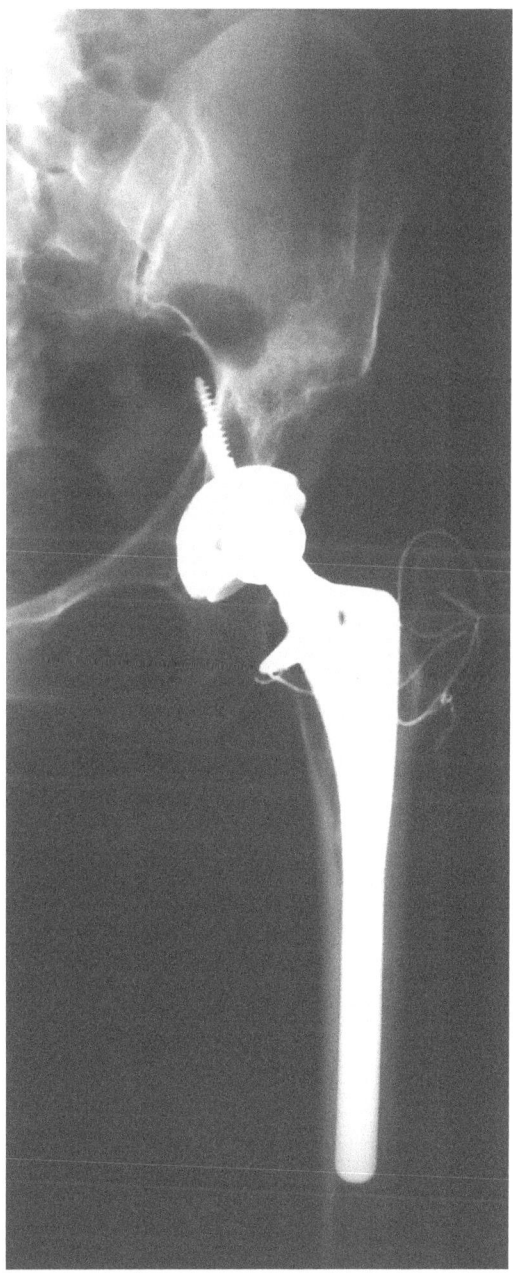

Fig. 4.49 Asymptomatic polyethylene wear was observed, 13 years after primary replacement. A polyethylene liner exchange was followed

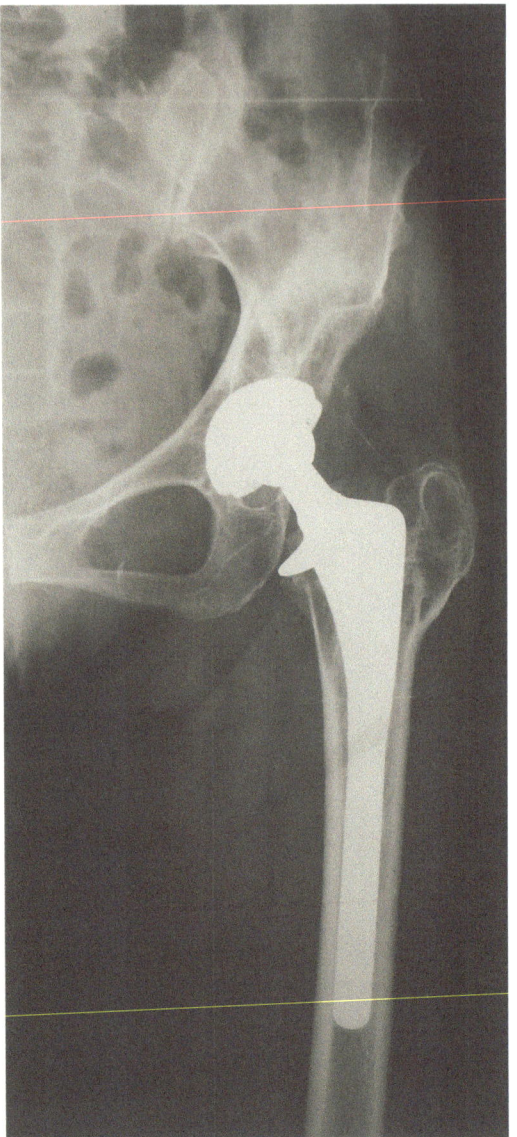

4.11   Case 11

This female patient was born in 1962 with complete dislocation of the left hip. She had no treatment in infancy. She was limping since then, and started to have hip pain around the age of 25 years. At the age of 28 years, in 1990, we operated her for C2 subtype high dislocation. A hybrid THR was performed. Even since then and for the next 26 years until the last follow-up, the patient has had a normal, fully active life without hip pain and only a slight limp, because of 2 cm leg-length discrepancy (Figs. 4.51–4.53).

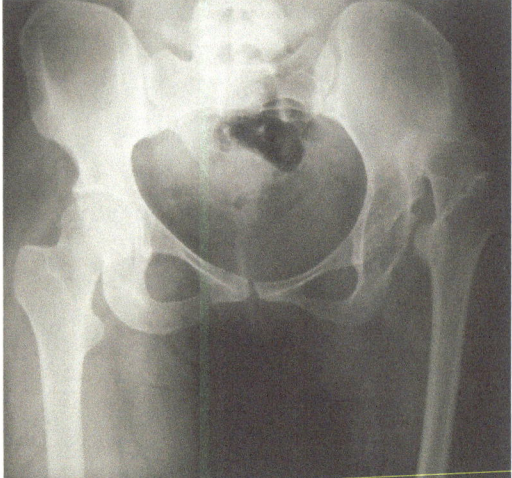

Fig. 4.51   Preoperative radiograph. There is a C1 subtype high dislocation of the left hip with 5 cm height

Fig. 4.50   The latest follow-up radiograph was taken 23 years after primary operation and 10 years after exchange of the polyethylene liner

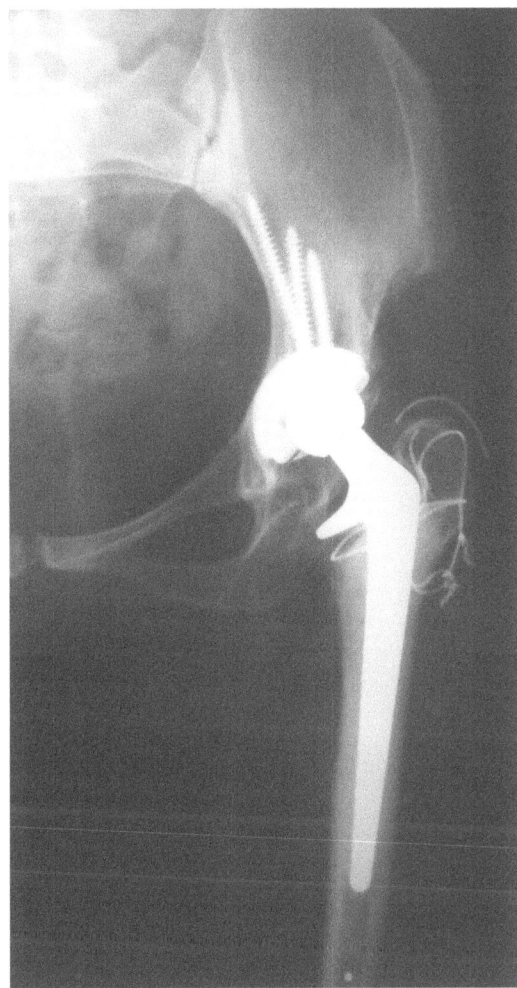

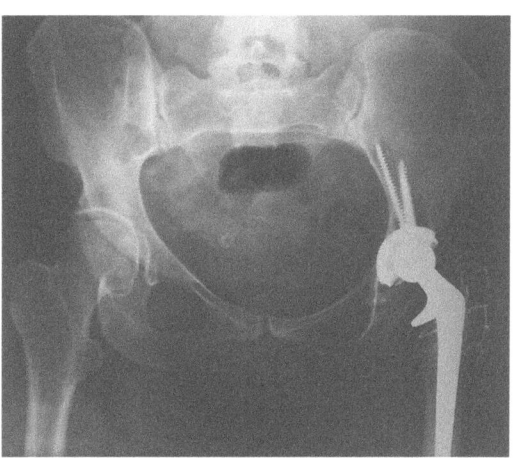

Fig. 4.53 The latest follow-up radiograph was taken 23 years postoperatively

Fig. 4.52 Radiograph taken 10 years postoperatively. One centimetre of femoral shortening was required at the time of surgery

Idiopathic Osteoarthritis

OA is the most common disease of the hip in adults. Two types of hip OA have been recognised: (a) idiopathic, when the underlying cause is unknown, and (b) secondary, when the predisposing cause is well defined. Furthermore, two main types of idiopathic OA have been described based on the direction of femoral head migration during the process of evolution of the degenerative changes: (a) eccentric, when superolateral or superomedial migration occurs, and (b) concentric, when medial, axial or global migration occurs.

Idiopathic OA occurs in patients of the middle age with normal hips since then. The natural history of the two main types differs radically. The eccentric type has a rapid deterioration, especially the superolateral type, while the concentric type has a considerably better prognosis, because deterioration is slow.

The most common cause of secondary OA is CHD. Selected cases with CHD from our registry are presented in the previous chapters.

5.1 Case 1

This female patient was born in 1922. In infancy, she was affected by poliomyelitis, and since then she was limping on the right leg. Pain in the left hip started around the age of 60 years and was rapidly deteriorating. The diagnosis of eccentric idiopathic OA was made, and in 1988 she underwent an LFA at the age of 66 years. Twenty-seven years postoperatively, she was 93 years old and had a pain-free hip and a good level of activity corresponding to her age. She was walking with a cane in the left hand because of previous poliomyelitis of the right limb (Figs. 5.1–5.7).

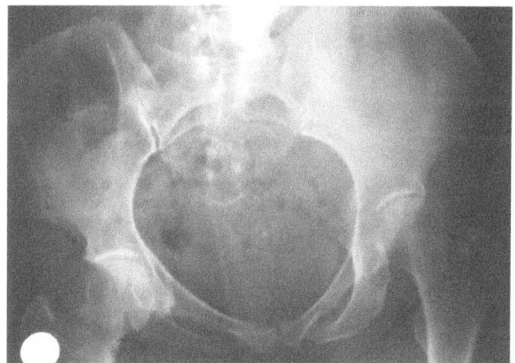

Fig. 5.1 Radiograph that was taken when the patient was 64 years old and had mild pain in the left hip because of eccentric idiopathic OA

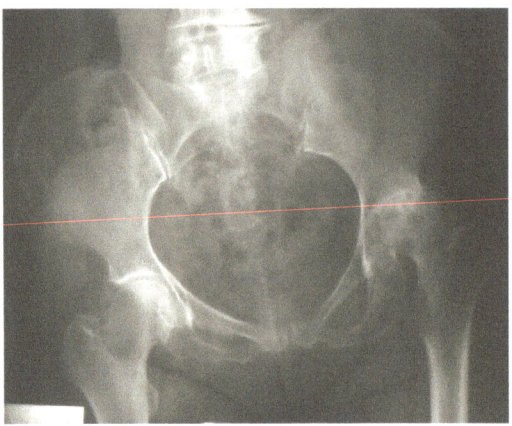

Fig. 5.2 There is remarkable deterioration of hip OA within 2 years

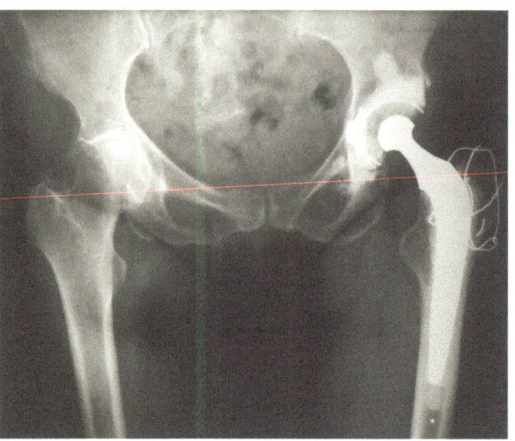

Fig. 5.5 Twenty years postoperatively

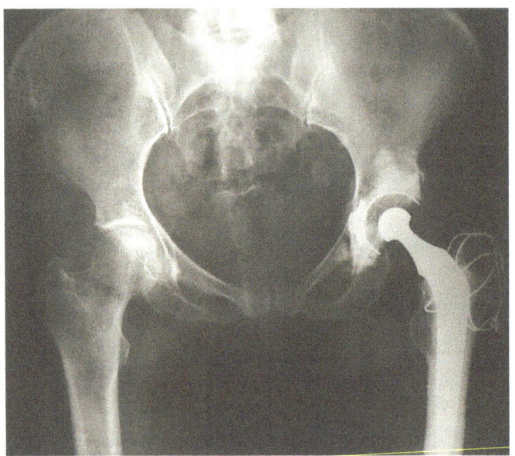

Fig. 5.3 An LFA of the left hip was performed, at the age of 66 years, in 1988

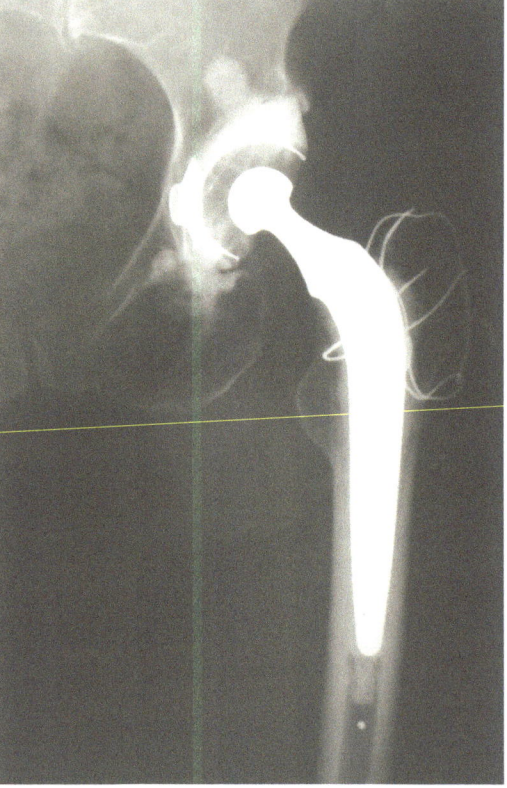

Fig. 5.6 The latest follow-up radiograph, 27 years post-operatively, when the patient was 93 years old

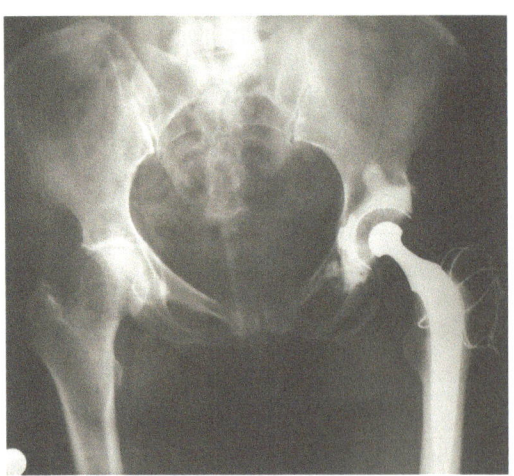

Fig. 5.4 The fifth-year follow-up radiograph

Fig. 5.7 In the meantime, deterioration of degenerative changes of the lumbar spine within 15 years was observed. Radiographs when the patient was (**a**) 78 years old and (**b**) 93 years old

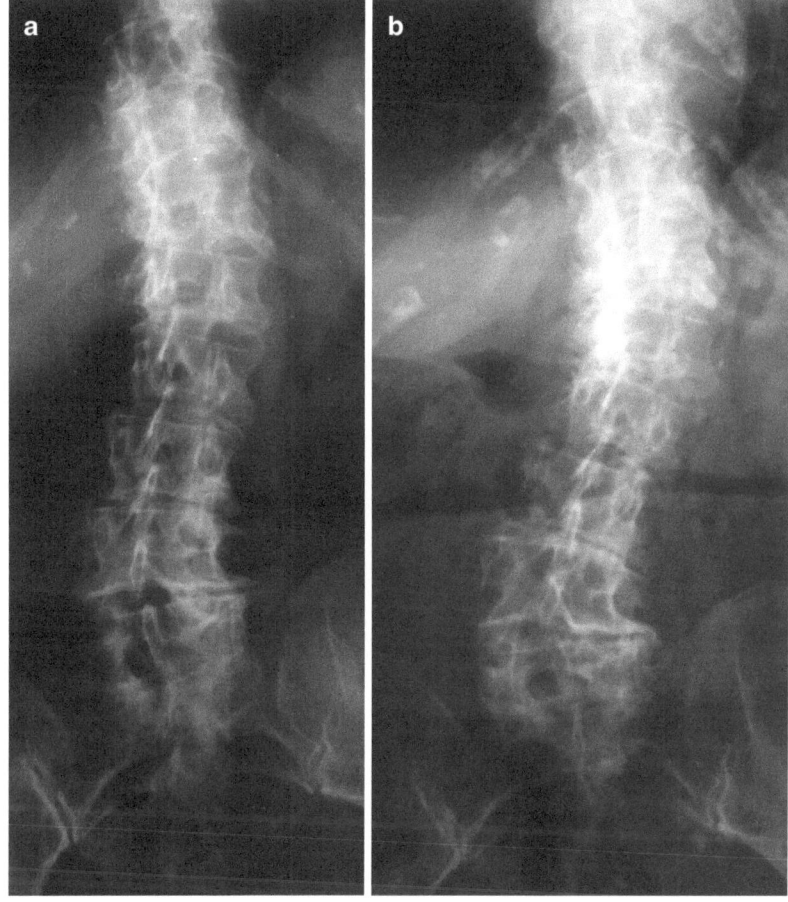

5.2   Case 2

This female patient was born in 1931. She had a normal life without hip pain until the age of 48 years, when eccentric idiopathic OA of the right hip had developed. LFA was performed in 1984, when the patient was 53 years old. One year later, pain in the contralateral hip started, also because of eccentric OA, and 8 years later in 1992, left LFA was followed. At the latest follow-up examination, the patient was 76 years old and she had normal activity level without pain in the hips (Figs. 5.8–5.12).

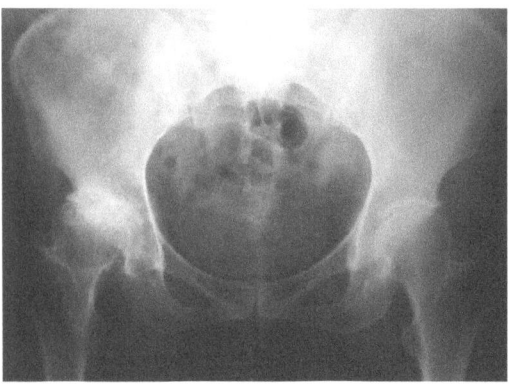

Fig. 5.8 This radiograph was taken in 1983, when the patient was 52 years old. She had increasing right hip pain for the last 4 years. Left hip was asymptomatic. LFA of the right hip was performed 1 year later

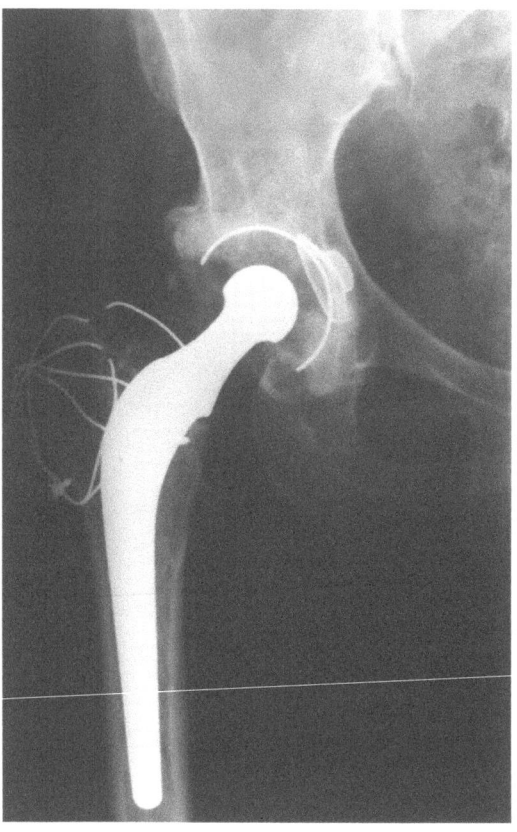

Fig. 5.9 In 1984, postoperative radiograph of the right hip

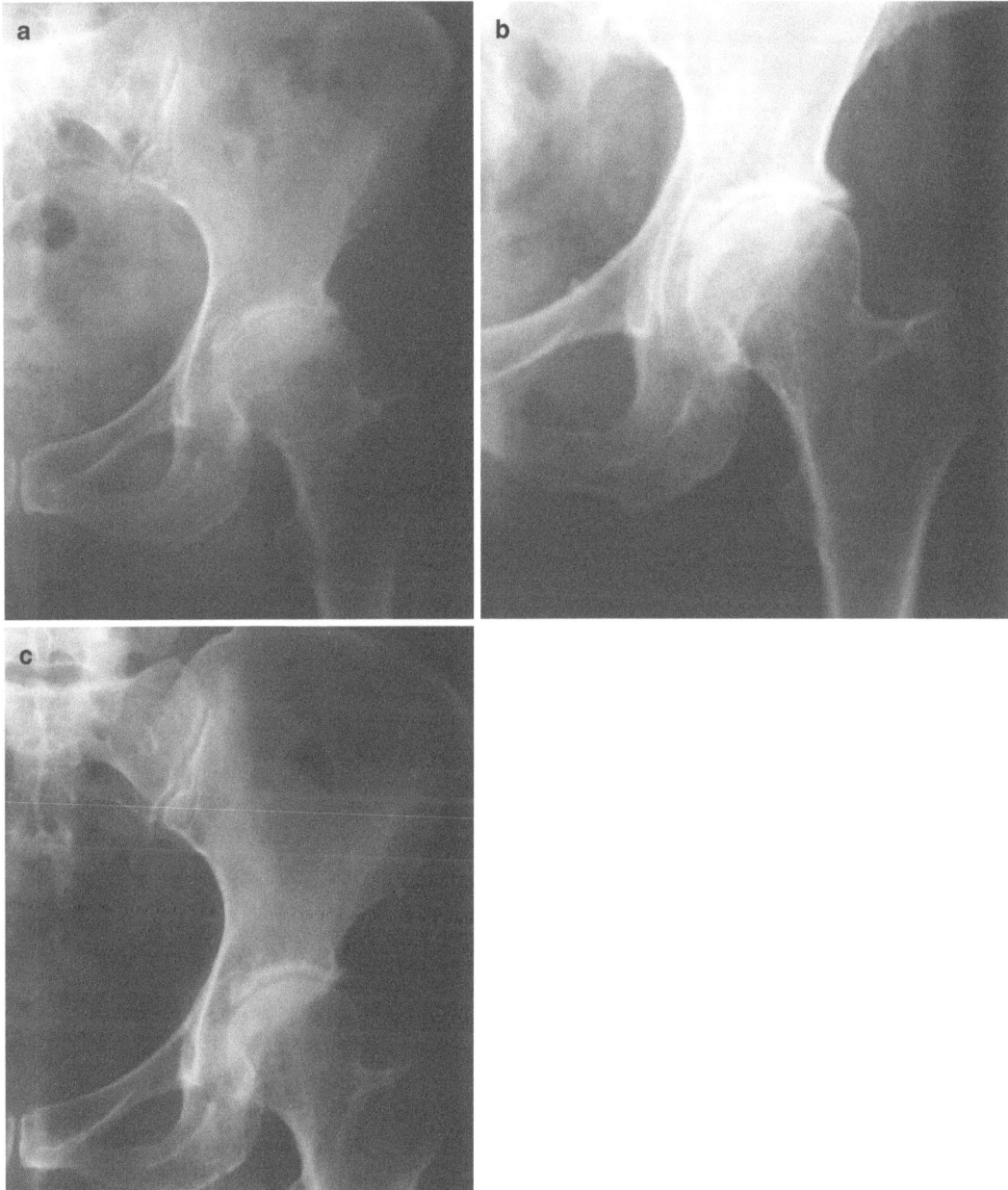

Fig. 5.10 There is a remarkable deterioration of the osteoarthritic changes of the left hip during the following years. Radiographs, at the age of (**a**) 54, when the hip symptoms had started, (**b**) 58 and (**c**) 61 years old. LFA was followed

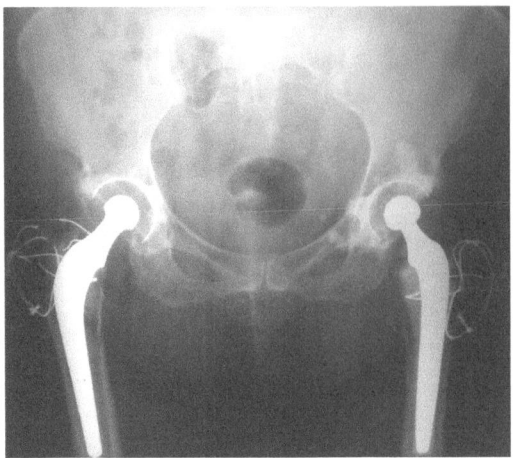

Fig. 5.11 Radiograph that was taken 18 years after LFA of the right hip and 10 years of the left

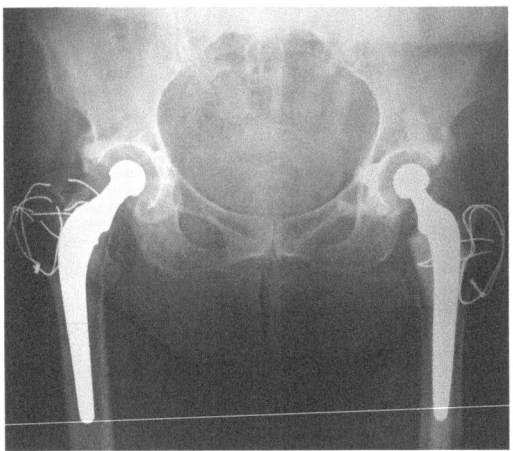

Fig. 5.12 The latest follow-up radiograph, 23 and 15 years after LFA of the right and left hip, respectively

5.3   Case 3

This female patient was born in 1926. She started having slight pain in the right hip at the age of 53 years and in the left at the age of 59 years. The diagnosis was concentric idiopathic OA of both hips. Deterioration of the degenerative changes was slow. LFA was performed in the right hip, when the patient was 63 years old in 1989, and in the left, 6 years later. The patient died, 90 years old, of reasons unrelated to the THRs, free of hip symptoms (Figs. 5.13–5.18).

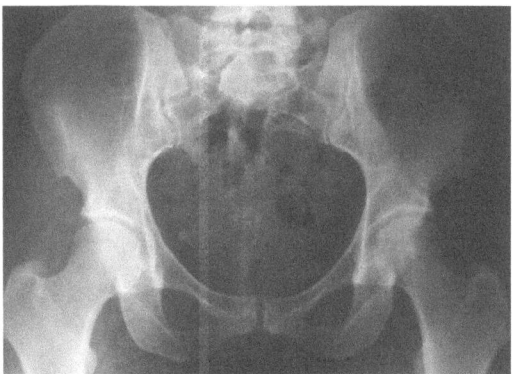

Fig. 5.13 Radiograph taken when the patient was 44 years old, in 1970, for reason unrelated to the hips (low back pain). Both hips were normal

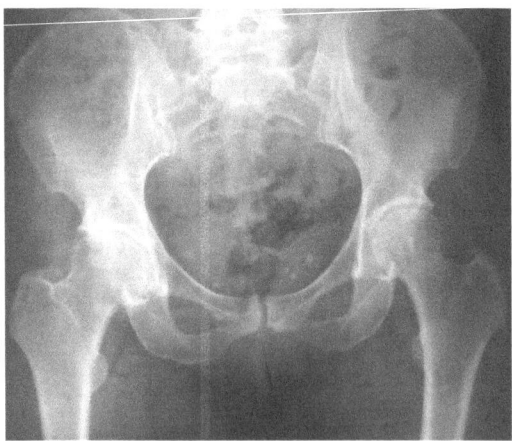

Fig. 5.14 Radiograph taken 16 years later, when the patient was 60 years old. Slight pain and limping had started 7 years previously in the right and 1 year previously in the left

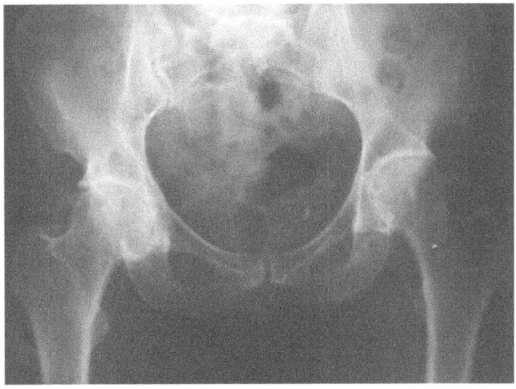

Fig. 5.15 Radiograph taken in 1989, before right THR

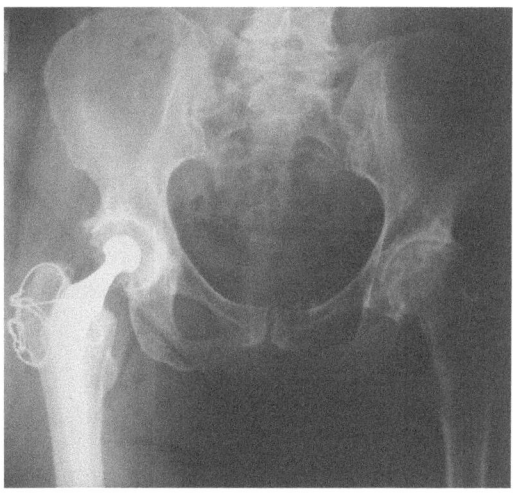

Fig. 5.17 Radiograph taken in 1995, 6 years after right THR, when the left THR was decided

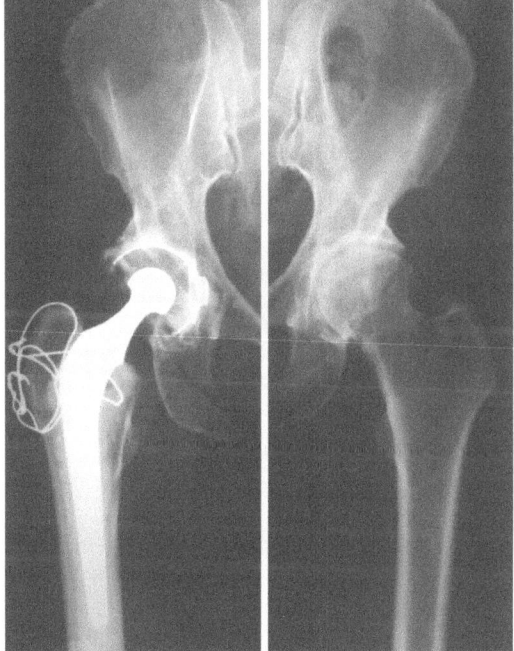

Fig. 5.16 One year after right THR. There is slow deterioration of the left hip OA

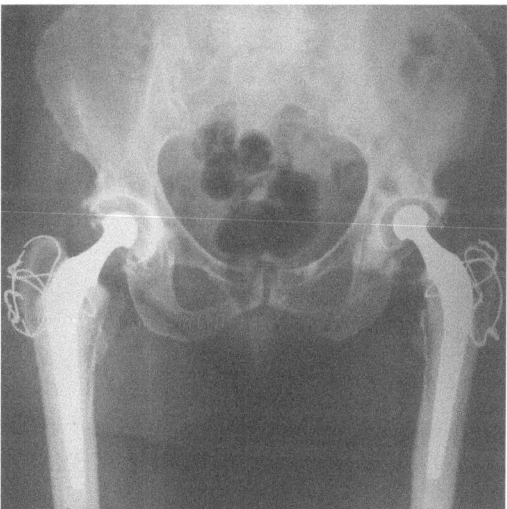

Fig. 5.18 The last follow-up radiograph, 21 and 15 years after right and left THR, respectively

5.4   Case 4

This female patient was born in 1922. She started having slight pain in the right hip around the age of 45 years and in the left around the age of 55 years, because of concentric OA. The deterioration was slow. LFA in the right hip was performed when she was 62 years old in 1984 and 6 years later in the left. The patient died at the age of 87 years, free of hip symptoms (Figs. 5.19–5.23).

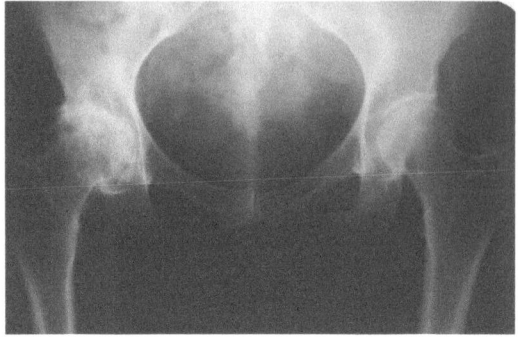

Fig. 5.21 Radiograph at the age of 62 years, when a right THR was performed

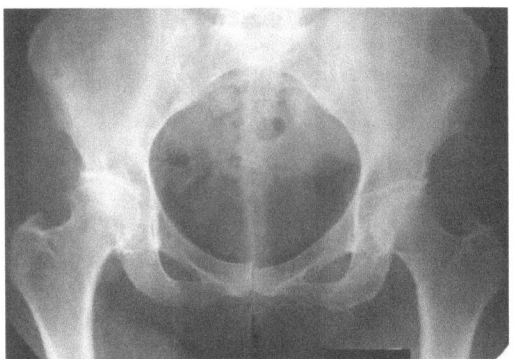

Fig. 5.19 Radiographs taken when the patient was 57 years old. She had symptoms of the right hip with duration of 12 years and of the left with duration of 2 years

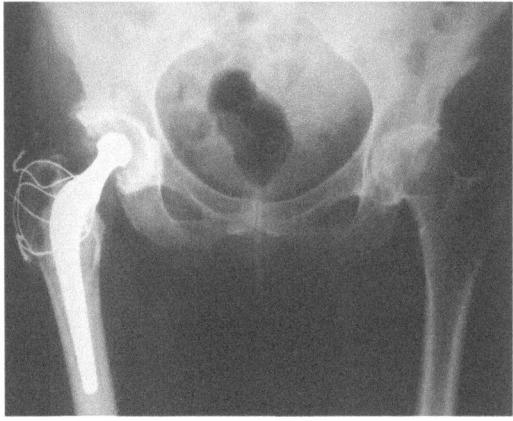

Fig. 5.22 Six years after right THR and before THR of the left hip

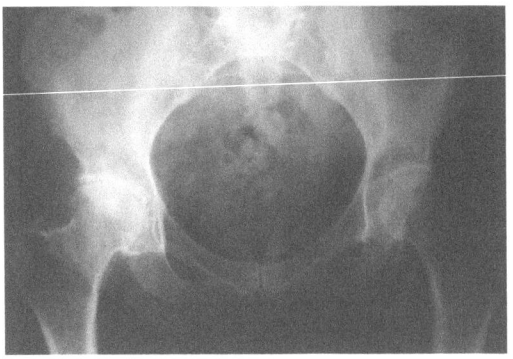

Fig. 5.20 Radiograph at the age of 60 years

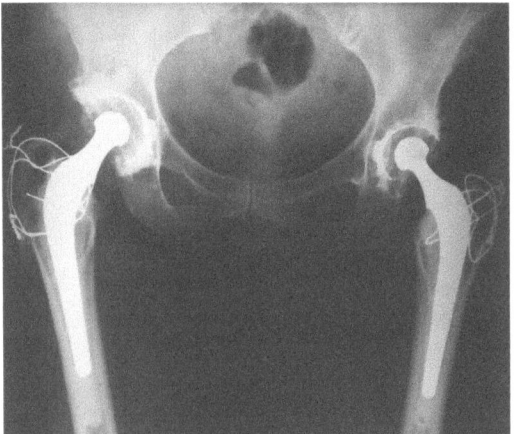

Fig. 5.23 The latest radiograph, when the patient was 82 years old, 20 and 14 years after right and left hip replacement, respectively

Inflammatory Arthritis

Inflammatory arthritis includes a group of systemic diseases such as rheumatoid arthritis, juvenile idiopathic arthritis, adult Still's disease, inflammatory bowel disease, ankylosing arthritis, systemic lupus and psoriatic arthritis. It is characterised by inflammation of the joints and is a common cause of severe hip involvement leading to THR. It affects young patients in the productive years of their life and usually involves multiple joints.

During the previous decades, patients with inflammatory arthritis, especially these with juvenile arthritis, usually needed a hip replacement before the age of 30 years. THR improves patients' pain and function, despite the multi-articular involvement and the fact that the biomechanical properties of soft tissues and bones are limited. Increased reoperation rate, and intraoperative, early and late post-operative complication rates, including infection and dislocation, in patients with inflammatory arthritis have been reported in the literature.

Patients with ankylosing arthritis, having mainly severe hips and spine problems, experience also impressive improvement of function after THR.

© Springer International Publishing AG 2017
K. Lampropoulou-Adamidou, G. Hartofilakidis, *Total Hip Replacement*,
DOI 10.1007/978-3-319-53360-5_6

6.1   Case 1

This male patient was born in 1957. He was diagnosed with juvenile idiopathic arthritis in childhood. He was referred to us at the age of 28 years. He was severely disabled; walking with both hips and knees in 30° fixed flexion having limited further flexion. In 1987, when the patient was 30 years old, we performed replacement of both hips and knees within 2 months. For THRs porous-coated anatomic (PCA) prostheses were used and for TKRs the Endo-Model® rotational knee prostheses were used. The patient gained full extension in both hips and knees, and functional painless motion for the next 27 years until 2014. After that period of productive years, he had a series of complications treated by our team in the next 2 years as followed:

- Periprosthetic fracture of the left femur just distal to the tip of the stem treated with open reduction and internal fixation
- Polyethylene liner wear of the right hip treated with exchange, in addition to revision of the acetabular shell, although the latter was well-fixed, because of unavailability of spare parts
- Polyethylene liner wear of the right TKR treated with exchange
- Periprosthetic fracture of the right femur just proximal to the tip of the TKR femoral component treated with open reduction and internal fixation

At the latest follow-up examination, in 2016, at the age of 59 years, he had almost full range of painless motion of hips and knees with acceptable level of activities, although he was limping heavily (Figs. 6.1–6.5).

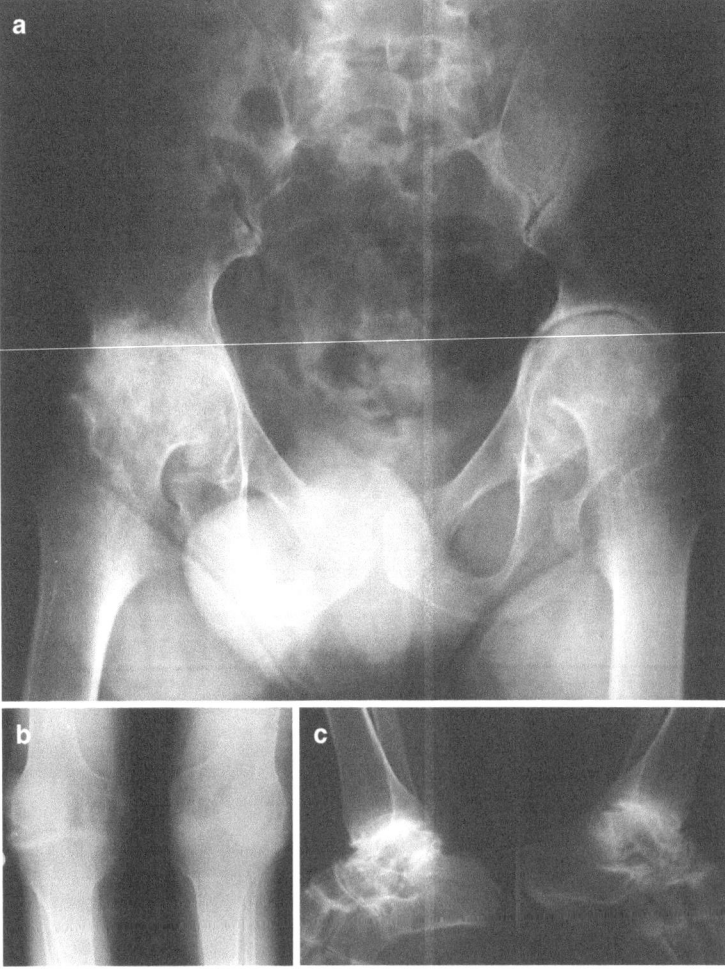

Fig. 6.1 Radiographs of (**a**) hips, (**b**) knees and (**c**) ankles when the patient was 30 years old

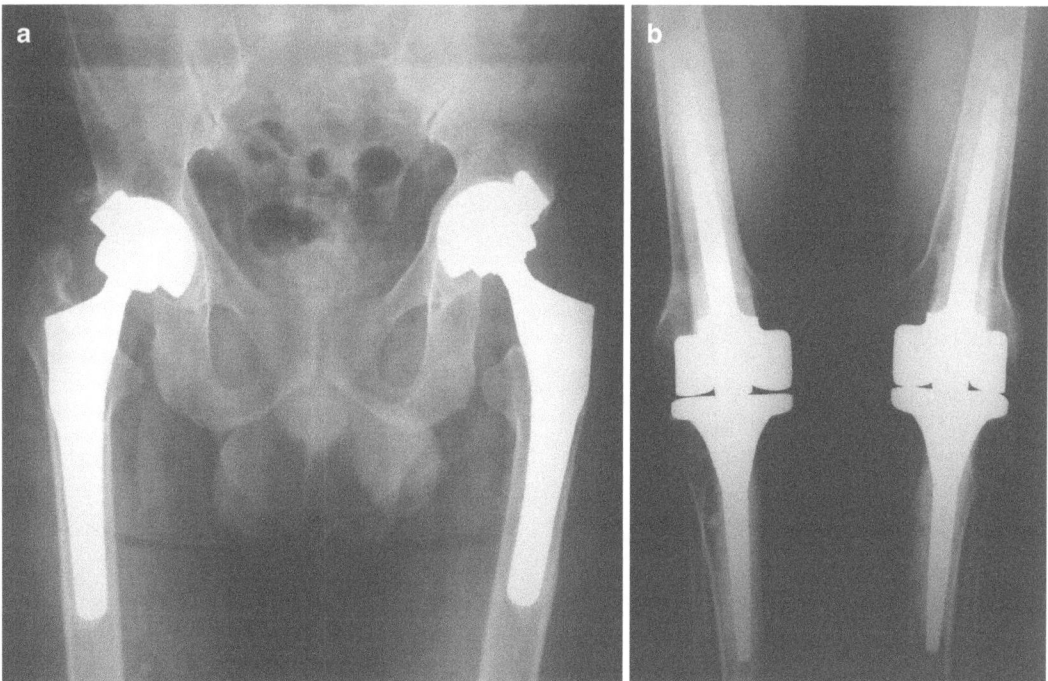

Fig. 6.2 Twelve years after reconstruction of (**a**) hips and (**b**) knees

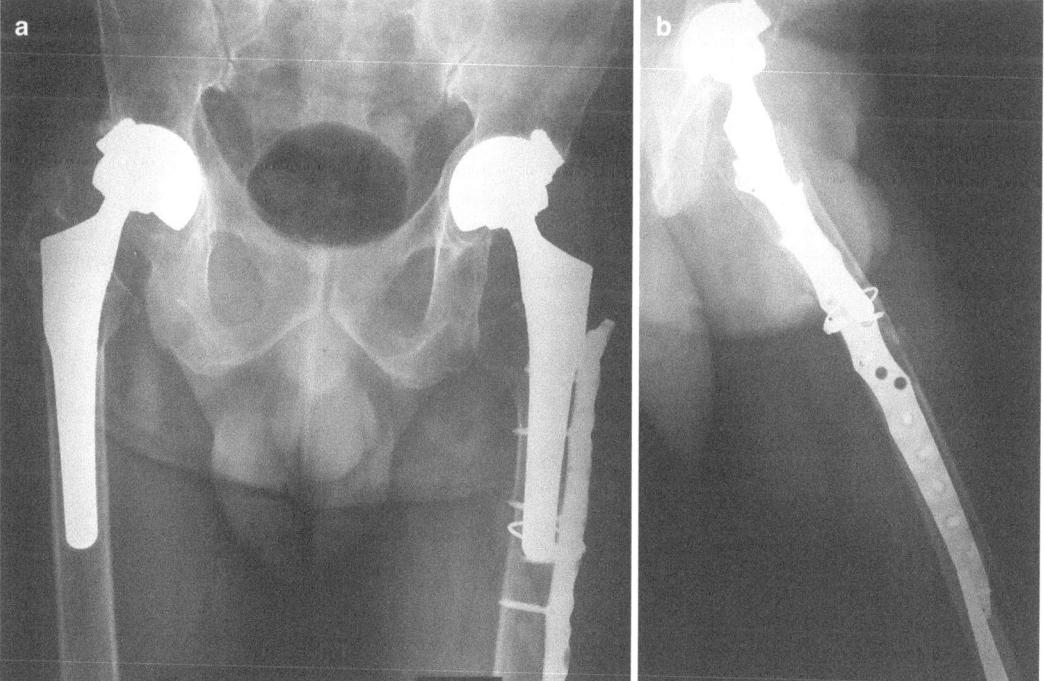

Fig. 6.3 (**a**) Anteroposterior and (**b**) lateral radiograph after internal osteosynthesis of the periprosthetic fracture of the left femur occurred 27 years after primary THR. There is also a significant wear of the right polyeth- ylene liner. Revision of the acetabular component in addi- tion to the polyethylene liner was followed 1 year later, because of unavailability of spare parts

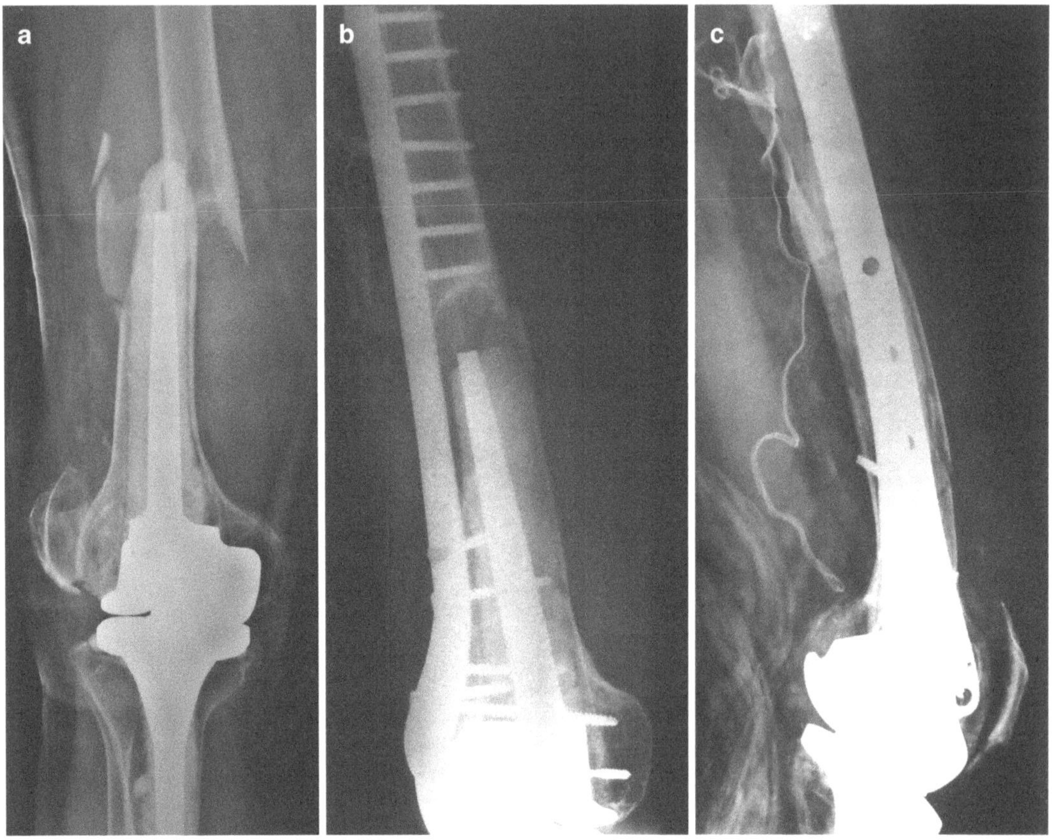

Fig. 6.4 Radiographs of (**a**) the right femur after the periprosthetic fracture treated with (**b**, **c**) open reduction and internal fixation

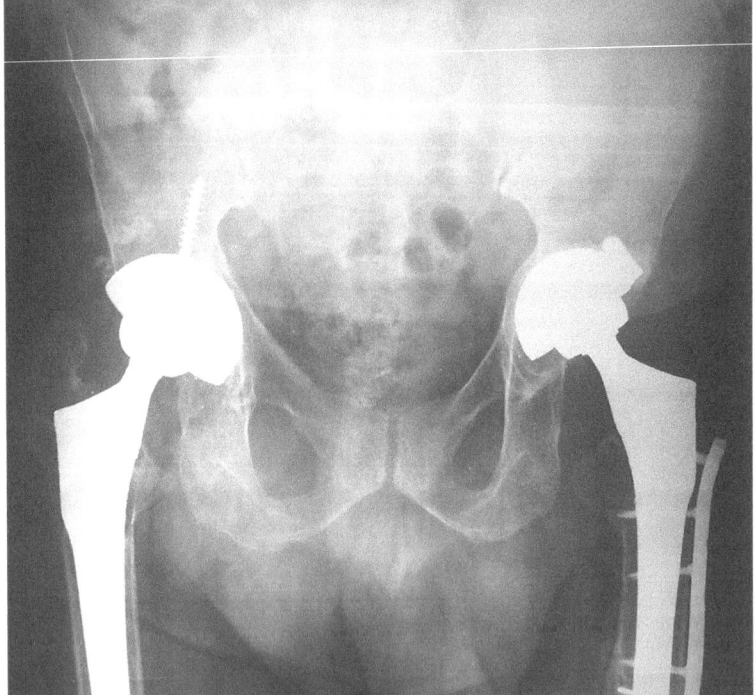

Fig. 6.5 The latest follow-up radiograph 29 years after primary THRs and 1 year after revision of the right acetabular component

6.2   Case 2

This female patient was born in 1949. She was diagnosed with rheumatoid arthritis at the age of 20 years. We operated her, in 1984, when she was 35 years old. LFA of both hips was performed. She was free of hip symptoms and she had normal activity for many years; however, a revision of the right cup was needed 19 years later, because of wear. At the latest follow-up, 32 years after primary THRs and 13 years after right acetabular component revision, she had symptomless hips and normal activity level (Figs. 6.6–6.10).

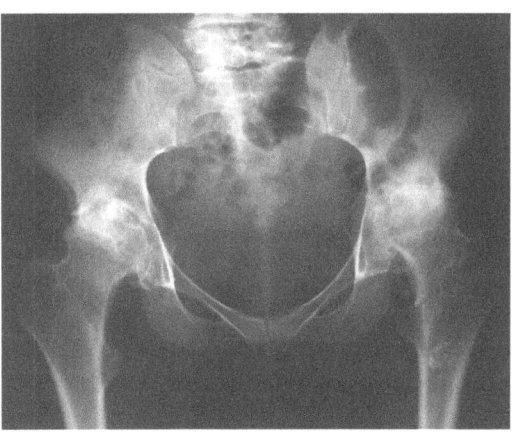

Fig. 6.6 Preoperative radiograph

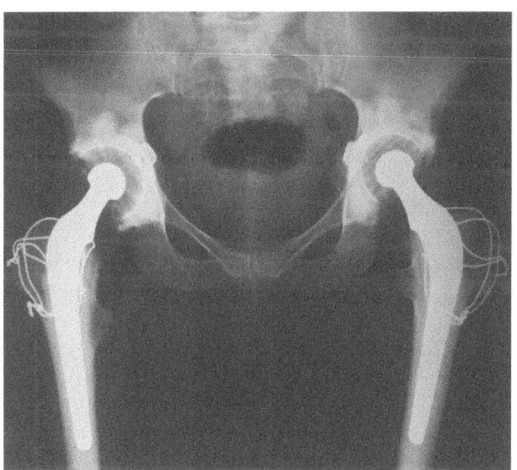

Fig. 6.7 Postoperative radiograph, when the patient was 35 years old

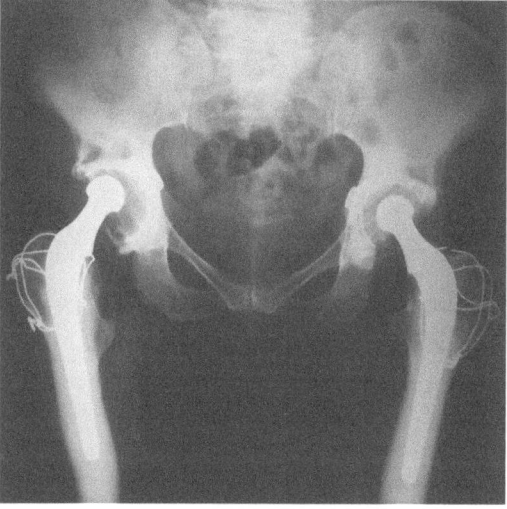

Fig. 6.8 Seventeen years postoperatively, symptomless wear of the right cup was noticed

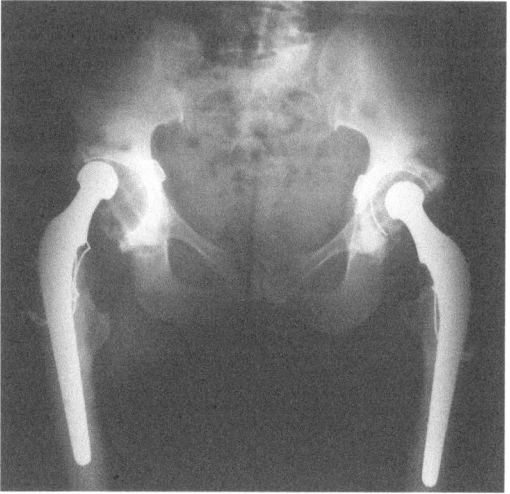

Fig. 6.9 Two years later, wear of the right cup had increased and its revision was decided. Slight wear of the left cup, present already since previous radiograph, had not progressed

Fig. 6.10 The latest follow-up radiograph, 32 years after primary THRs and 13 years after revision of the right acetabular component

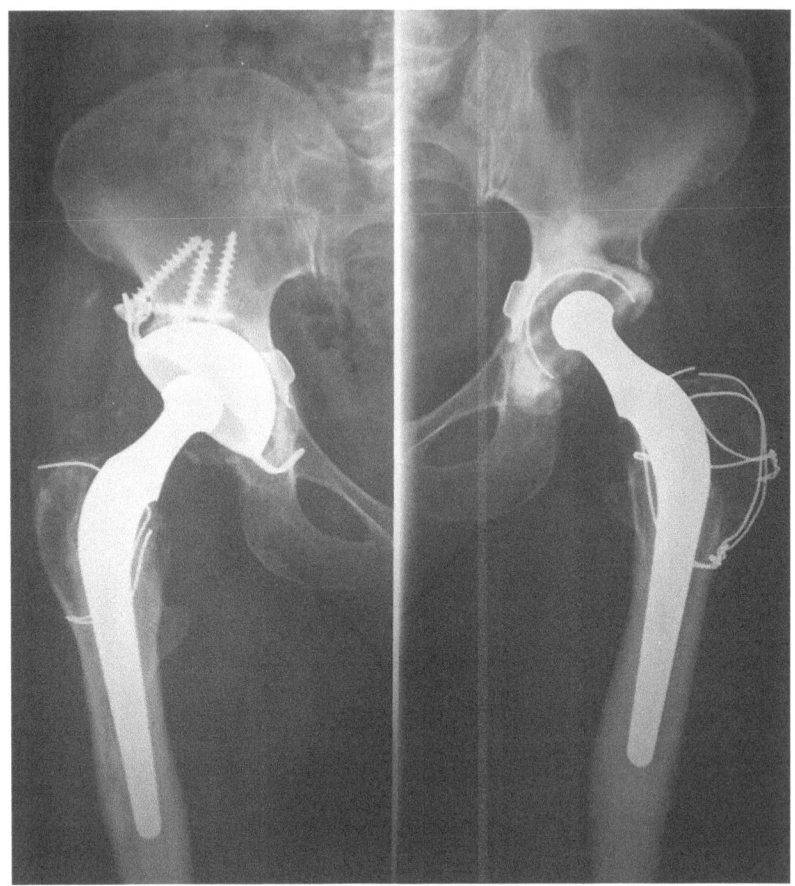

6.3   Case 3

This male patient was born in 1950. He was diag-nosed with ankylosing spondylitis at the age of 18 years. He underwent by us left LFA, when he was 29 years old in 1979, and 9 years later, right LFA. Revision of the left cup was performed 26 years after primary THR in 2005 and of the right cup 18 years after primary THR in 2006. At the last follow-up examination, the patient was 66 years old, free of hip pain, and had a normal activity level (Figs. 6.11–6.15).

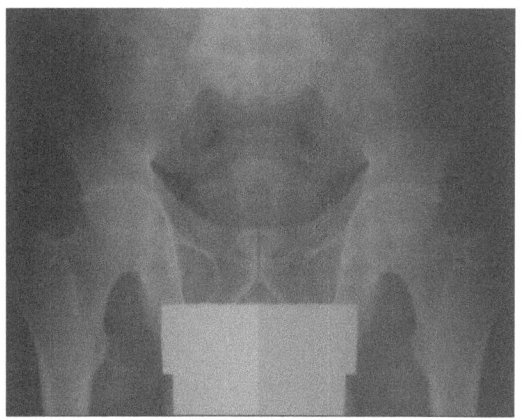

Fig. 6.11 Preoperative radiograph taken in 1979. The patient had severe pain and stiffness from the neck down to the lower back and both hips

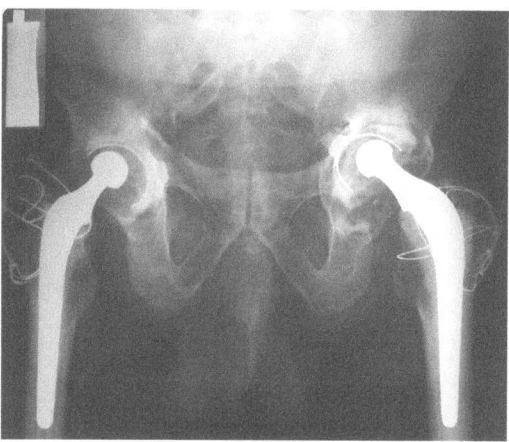

Fig. 6.13 Eight years later, wear of the cup had increased in both hips. Revision of both acetabular components was followed within 1 year

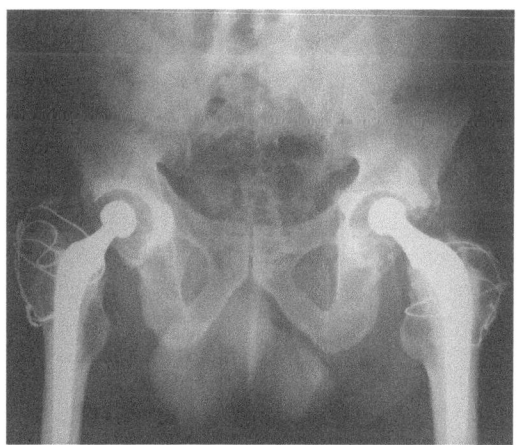

Fig. 6.12 Radiograph taken in 1996, 17 years after LFA of the left hip and 8 years of the right. Polyethylene wear, especially in the left hip, was noticed

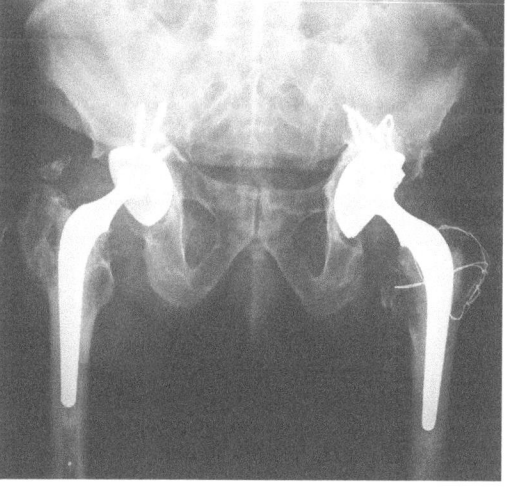

Fig. 6.14 The latest follow-up radiograph was taken 11 and 10 years after revision of the acetabular components and 37 and 26 years after primary implantation of femoral components of the left and right hip, respectively

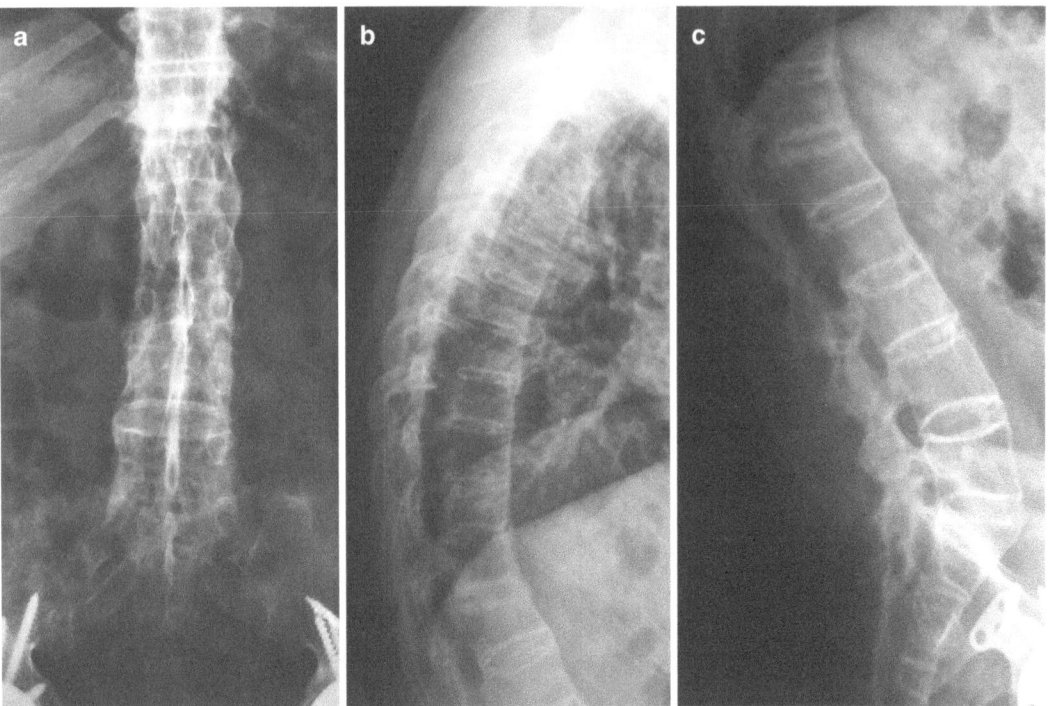

Fig. 6.15 (**a**) Anteroposterior radiograph of the lumbar spine and (**b**, **c**) lateral radiographs of the thoracic and lumbar spine that were taken at the patient's latest follow-up. Asymptomatic complete fusion is present

6.4   Case 4

This female patient was born in 1968. She was diagnosed with juvenile idiopathic arthritis at the age of 16 years. We first examined the patient, when she was 25 years old, in 1993. She had great disability, with severe pain and great limitation of motion in both hips. We considered THRs as the only solution. At the eighth-year-postoperative evaluation, polyethylene wear and extensive osteolysis around acetabular compo-

nents, more pronounced in the left, were noticed. The patient was asymptomatic and refused the recommended exchange of both liners. During the following years, osteolysis was increasing. She became symptomatic 6 years later, in 2007, whereupon she accepted to undergo revision of both acetabular components. At that time, more complicated techniques were needed. At the latest follow-up evaluation, she was 48 years old, free of hip pain and she had normal activity level (Figs. 6.16–6.21).

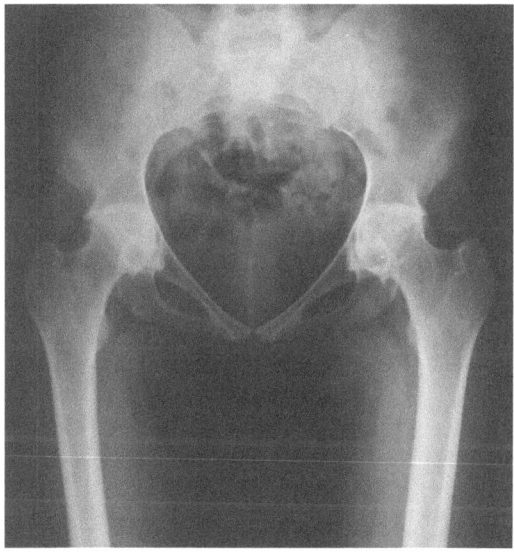

Fig. 6.16 Preoperative radiograph in 1993. Bilateral cementless THRs were followed in 20 days interval

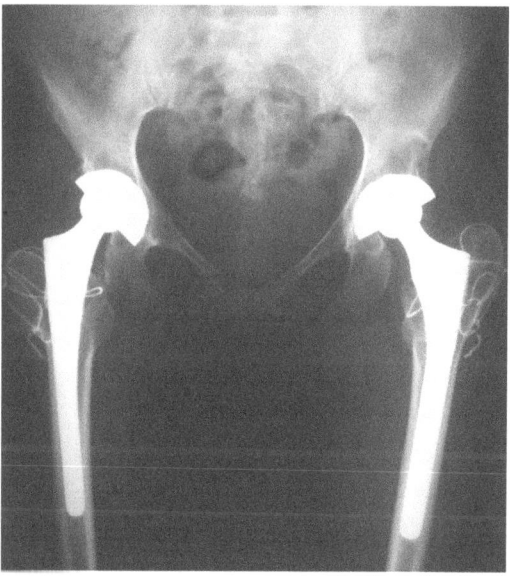

Fig. 6.18 Radiograph taken at the seventh postoperative year. Polyethylene wear and osteolysis around both acetabular components, more pronounced in the left, were observed

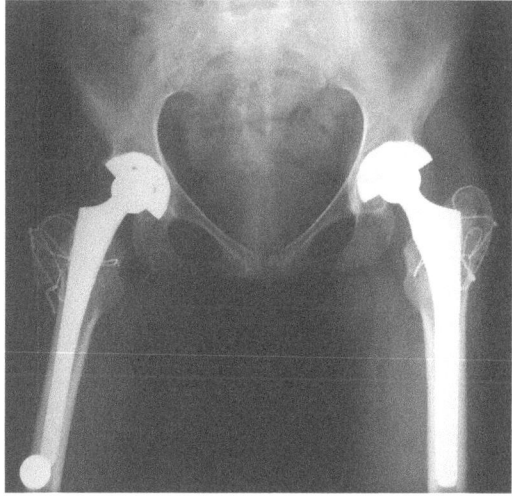

Fig. 6.17 Six months postoperatively

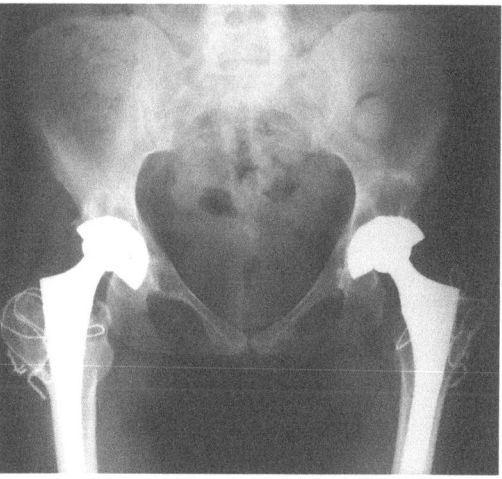

Fig. 6.19 Eleven years postoperatively, there was increase of polyethylene liner wear and osteolysis. The patient refused our recommendation for liner exchange

Fig. 6.20 The 14th postoperative year (**a**) anteroposterior and (**b**, **c**) lateral radiographs of both hips revealed that osteolysis around both acetabular components had significantly increased. At that time, the patient became symptomatic and accepted revision of both acetabular components

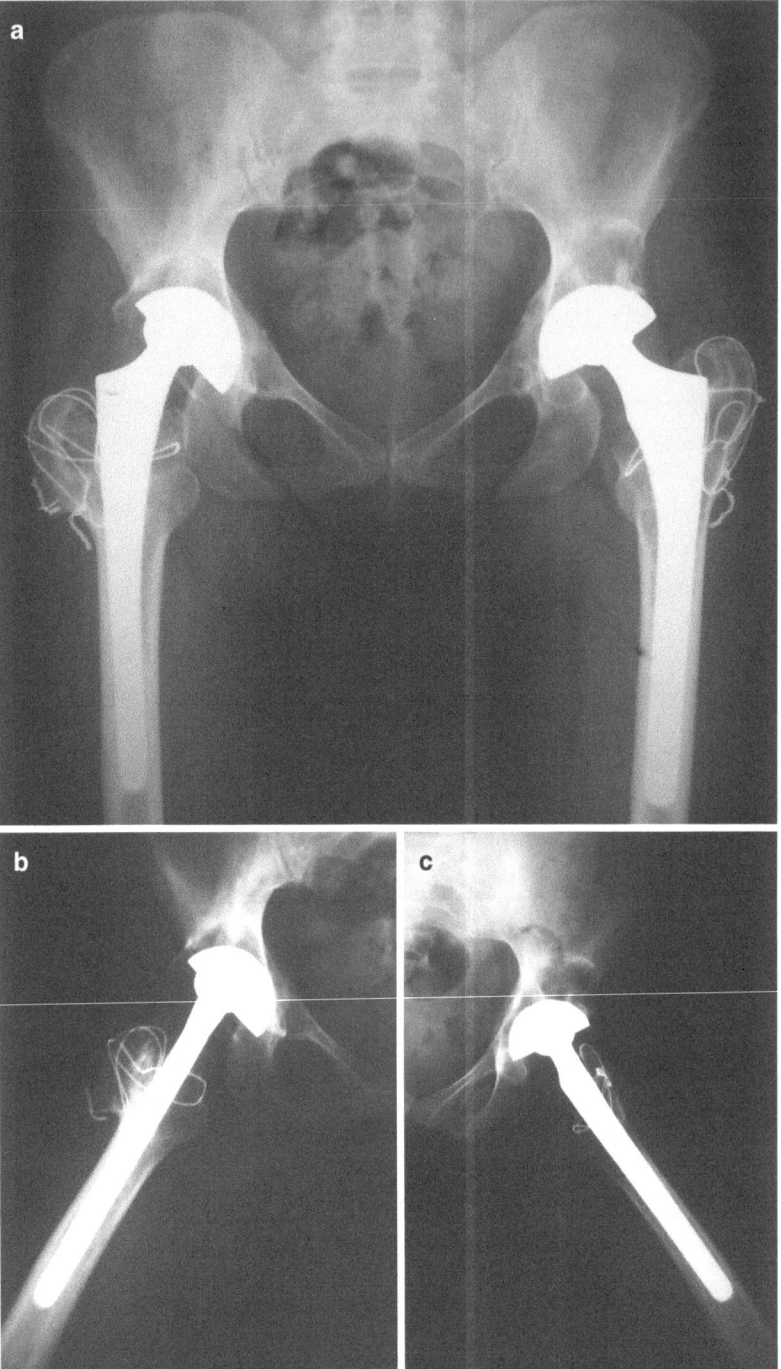

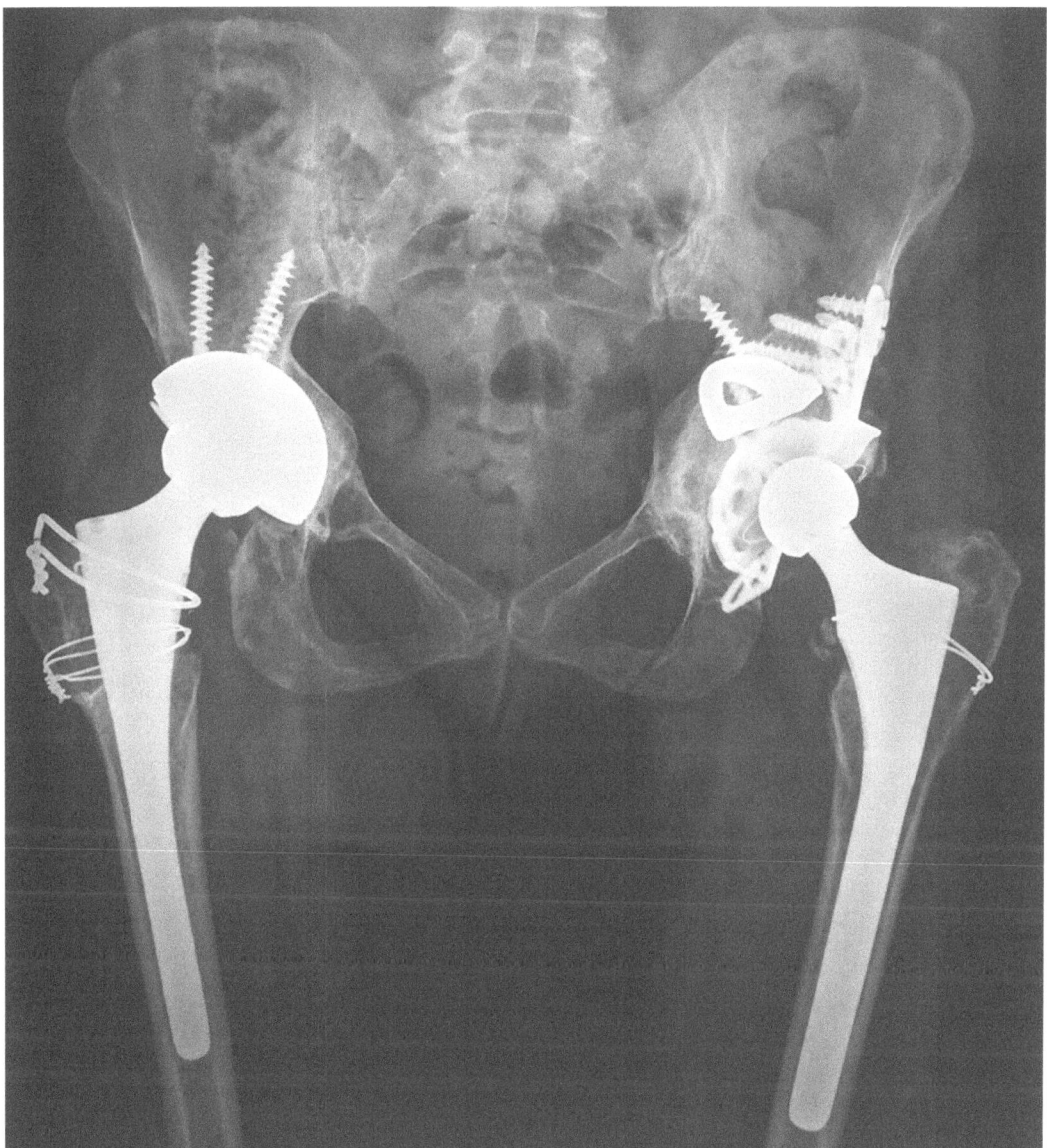

Fig. 6.21 The last radiograph was taken 7 and 6 years after revision of the left and right acetabular components, respectively, and 21 years after primary implantation of the femoral components

Avascular Necrosis of the Femoral Head

Avascular necrosis (AVN) or osteonecrosis of the femoral head is characterised by cellular death and subsequent femoral head collapse caused by interruption of bone blood supply. It affects young adults, usually in the third and fourth decade of their life. Bilateral hip involvement reached up to 80% within 2 years. Direct causes of AVN include trauma, haematologic diseases (haemoglobinopathies, leukaemia, lymphoma), dysbaric disorders and storage disorders (Gaucher's disease), and indirect causes include coagulation disorders, alcohol abuse, smoking, pregnancy, steroids (endogenous or exogenous), systemic lupus erythematosus and organ transplantation. When the underlying cause of AVN is not well defined, the diagnosis of idiopathic AVN is considered. Despite the young age of patients, THR remains the only method of treatment for the advanced stages of the disease.

We selected two cases of idiopathic osteonecrosis and two cases of sickle cell disease, which is not uncommon in our country. The cases of idiopathic osteonecrosis include the presentation of two sisters with bilateral hip involvement. An extended laboratory examination was performed in the older sister, because of the unusual familial involvement which failed to reveal any abnormality.

Of note, a patient with sickle cell disease had a rare complication, unrelated with the diagnosis, 13 years after primary LFA. A broken wire migrated from the greater trochanter, causing severe trauma to the femoral artery.

© Springer International Publishing AG 2017
K. Lampropoulou-Adamidou, G. Hartofilakidis, *Total Hip Replacement*,
DOI 10.1007/978-3-319-53360-5_7

7.1   Case 1

This female patient was born in 1962. Hip pain and limping started at the age of 12 years. We first examined her, when she was 22 years old. AVN of both hips was diagnosed. THR was postponed since the age of 29 years in 1991. Hybrid THR was performed in both hips within 5 months. Left polyethylene liner exchange was performed 13 years postoperatively, in 2004, because of excessive polyethylene wear. Six months later, right acetabular component was also revised because of aseptic loosening. In the present, 25 years after primary operations, the patient is 54 years old and has asymptomatic hips and normal activities.

Of note, we could not identify any known causative factor of AVN, as well as laboratory examination for sickle cell disease (haemoglobin S [Hb S]), subtle coagulation disturbances (complete blood count [CBC], prothrombin time [PT] and international normalised ratio [INR], activated partial thromboplastin time [aPTT], anti-thrombin III [ATIII], activated protein C resistance [APC-R], protein C, protein S, fibrinogen and D-dimmer), autoimmune disorders, rheumatoid arthritis and systemic lupus erythematosus (SLE) (RA test, antinuclear antibody [ANA], anti-double stranded DNA [anti-dsDNA], complement component 3 [C3c], complement component 4 [C4], serum immunoelectrophoresis, C-reactive protein [CRP] and erythrocyte sedimentation rate [ESR]) and autoimmune thyroid diseases (thyroid-stimulating hormone [TSH], anti-thyroid peroxidase [anti-TPO] and anti-thyroglobulin [anti-Tg]) failed to reveal any abnormality (Figs. 7.1–7.6).

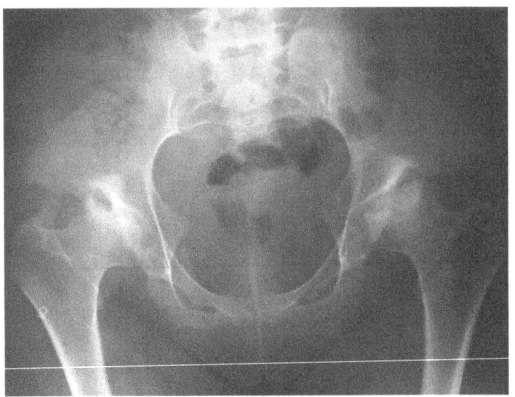

Fig. 7.1 Radiograph at the age of 22 years

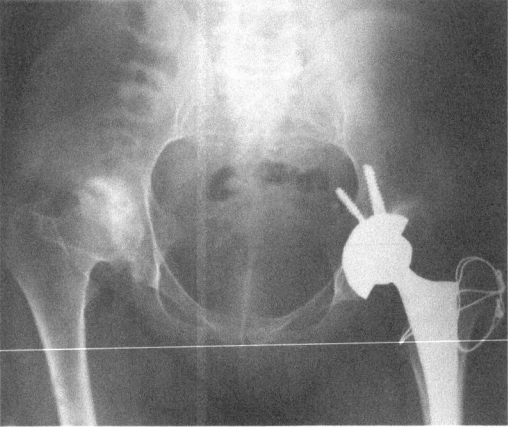

Fig. 7.3 Five months after left THR

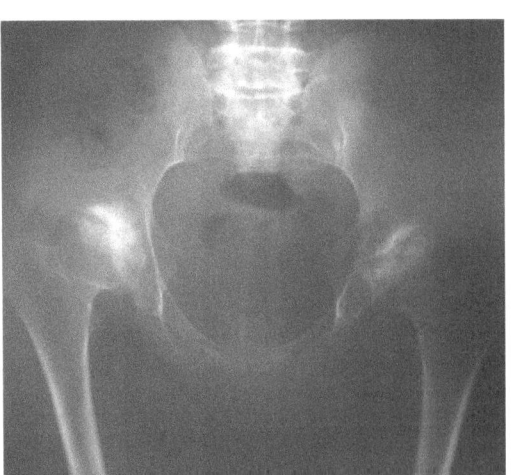

Fig. 7.2 Radiograph when THR was decided at the age of 29 years, in 1991

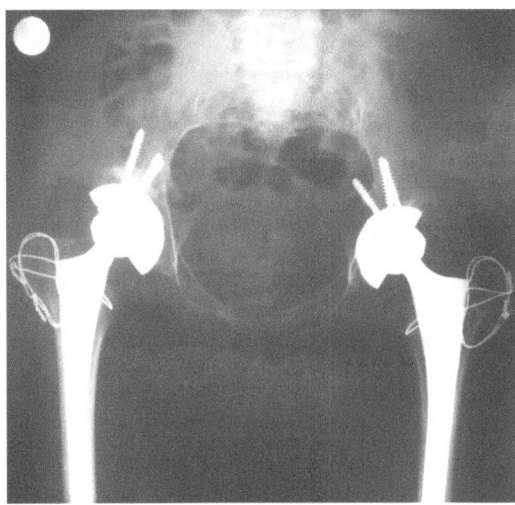

Fig. 7.4 This radiograph was taken 1 year after left THR and 7 months after right

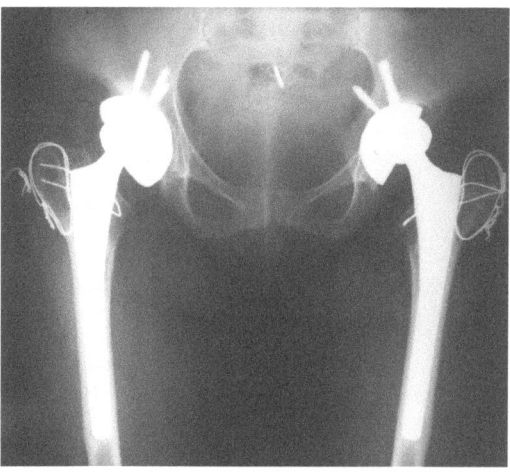

Fig. 7.5 Thirteen years postoperatively, excessive polyethylene wear of the left hip led to polyethylene liner exchange. Six months later, right acetabular component revision because of aseptic loosening was also needed

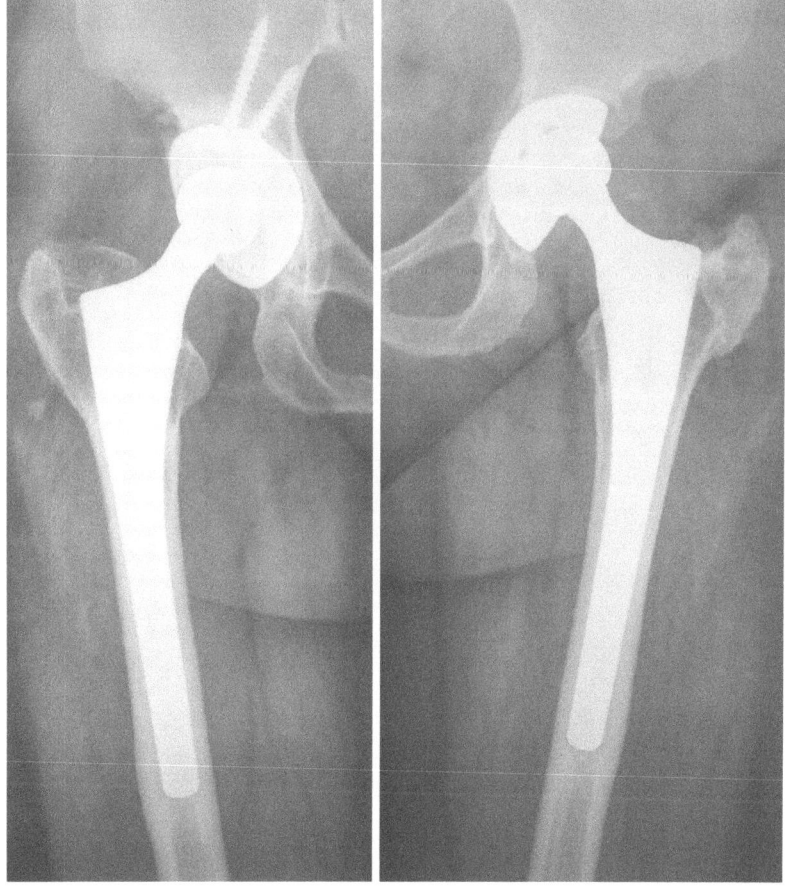

Fig. 7.6 The latest radiograph, 12 years after left polyethylene exchange and right acetabular component revision and 25 years after primary THRs

7.2   Case 2

This female patient, the sister of the patient described in the previous case, was born in 1967. Hip pain and limping started at the age of 12 years. We first examined her, when she was 26 years old.

ANV of both hips was diagnosed. THR was postponed since the age of 29. A hybrid THR was performed in 1996 in both hips within 6 weeks. In the present, 20 years after primary operations, the patient is 50 years old and has asymptomatic hips and normal activity (Figs. 7.7–7.12).

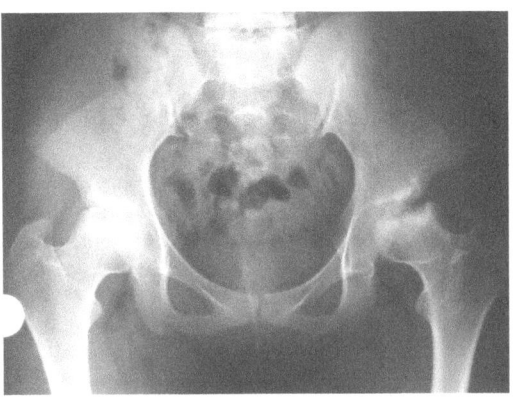

Fig. 7.7   Radiograph, when the patient was 14 years old

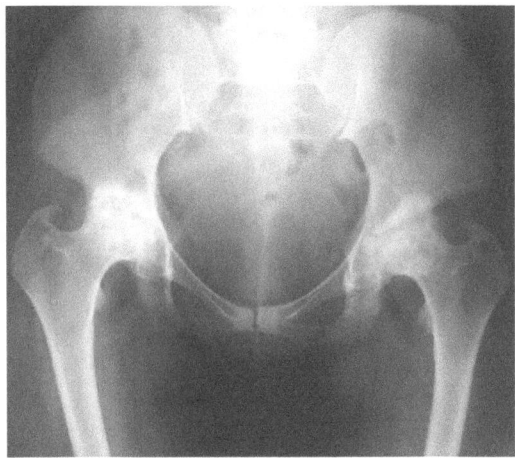

Fig. 7.9   Preoperative radiograph, when she was 29 years old

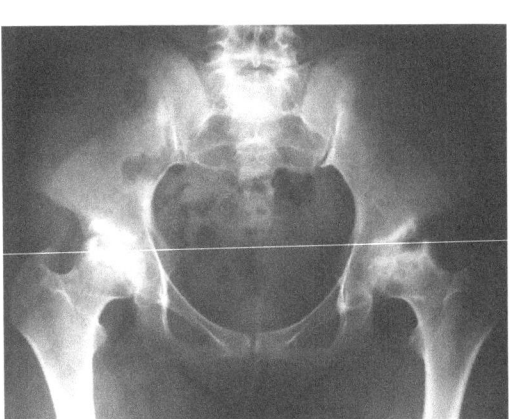

Fig. 7.8   Radiograph at the age of 18 years

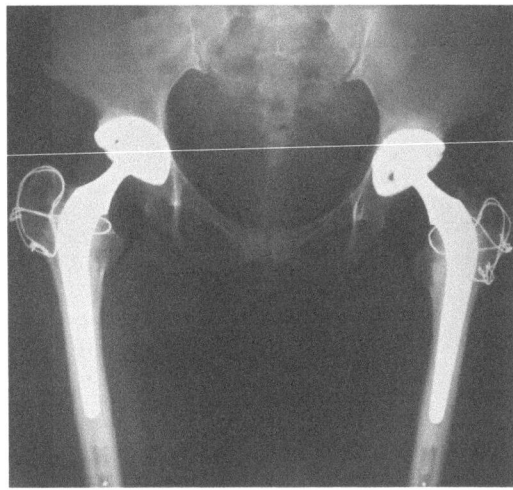

Fig. 7.10   Two years postoperatively

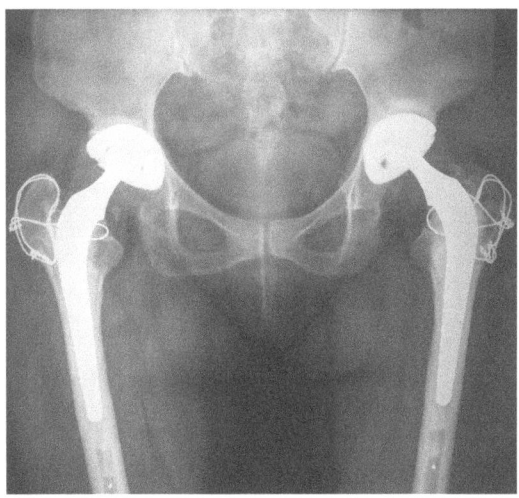

Fig. 7.11   Ten years after THRs

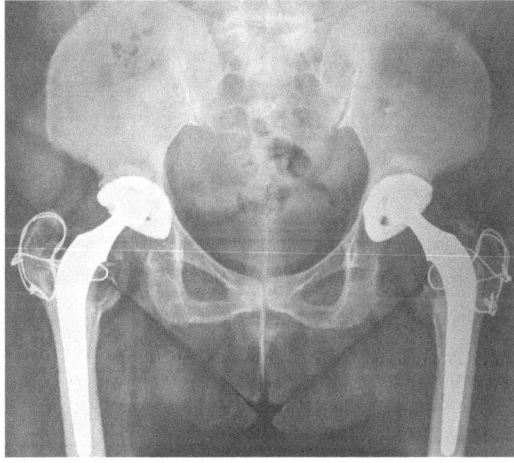

Fig. 7.12   Twenty years postoperatively

7.3   Case 3

This female patient was born in 1945. She had been diagnosed with sickle cell disease. She started to have pain in both hips and limping at the age of 28 years. ANV of the femoral heads was diagnosed. We performed left and right LFA when she was 30 and 31 years old, respectively. Revision of the right acetabular component because of aseptic loosening, 8 years after primary replacement, was performed.

Five years later, in 1989, she had a local ischaemic episode affecting her right leg. Arteriography revealed thrombosis of the right femoral artery. During vascular operation performed by a specialised surgeon, a migrated broken wire, from the previous THR, was found to pass through the artery. This case was published by Dayantas et al. in 1991 and remains unique until now.

The following years, the patient underwent revision of both components of the right hip and of the left cup. She died at the age of 62 years in a bad general condition because of sickle cell disease's complications (Figs. 7.13–7.16).

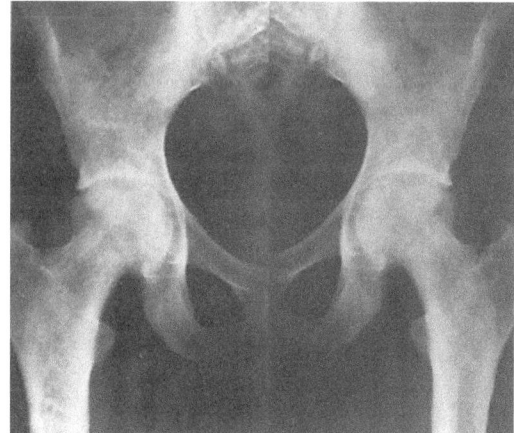

Fig. 7.13   Preoperative radiograph

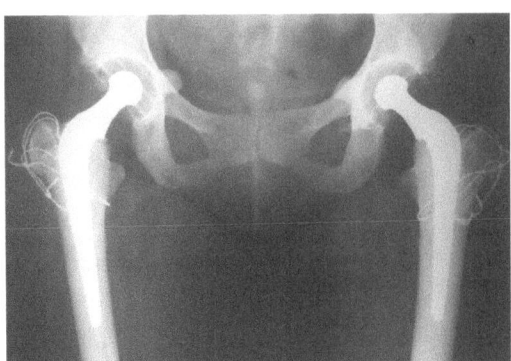

Fig. 7.14 Early postoperative radiograph

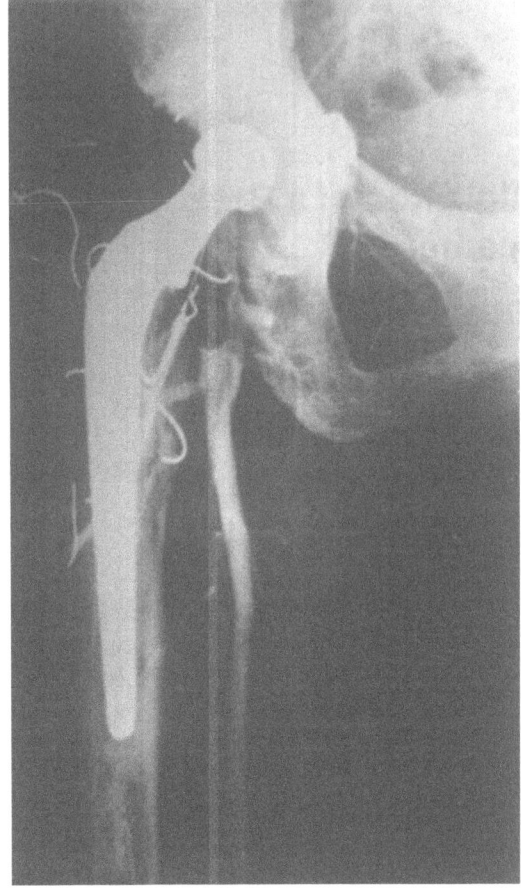

Fig. 7.15 Arteriography, when the patient had the ischaemic episode, revealed thrombosis of the right common
femoral artery causing significant stenosis and peripheral
emboli in the crural arteries. A migrated broken wire,
from the previous THR, was found to pass through the
artery

Fig. 7.16 The latest
follow-up radiograph:
(**a**) of the right hip,
30 years after primary
LFA, the right cup had
two previous revisions
and the stem one, and
(**b**) of the left hip,
31 years after primary
LFA, the cup had one
previous revision and
the stem is the original
one

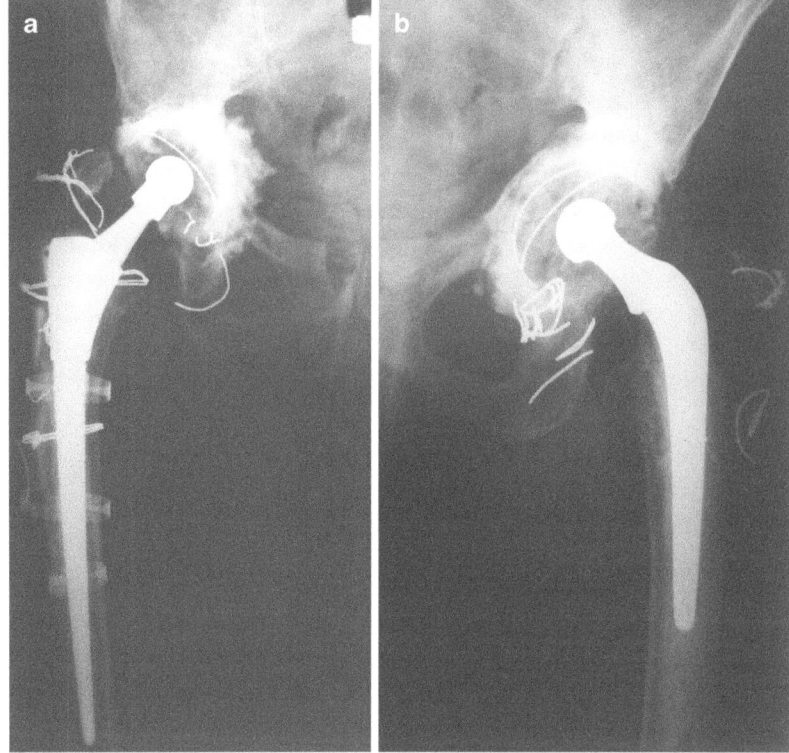

7.4   Case 4

This female patient was born in 1971. She had been diagnosed with sickle cell disease. Right hip pain and limping started at the age of 15 years and AVN of the right femoral head was diagnosed. Rapid clinical and radiographic deterioration made THR necessary, when the patient was 17 years old. Eleven years after surgery, both components' revision was needed because of aseptic loosening. Removal of the stem was performed with great difficulty using a "window" in the lateral cortex of the femur. A transverse fracture occurred at the level of the "window", during the last stages of the operation. The new femoral prosthesis, Charnley Elite long stem, and the prolonged use of crutches led to the healing of the fracture. Ten years later, re-revision of the acetabular component was performed, because of aseptic loosening.

At the last follow-up assessment, 7 years after the latter cup revision and 17 years after the intraoperative femoral fracture, the patient was 45 years old, free of hip symptoms and without limping and had normal activity level (Figs. 7.17–7.22).

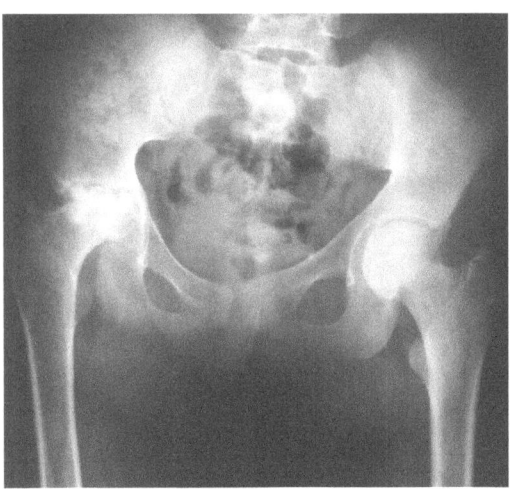

Fig. 7.17 Preoperative radiograph, when the patient was 17 years old

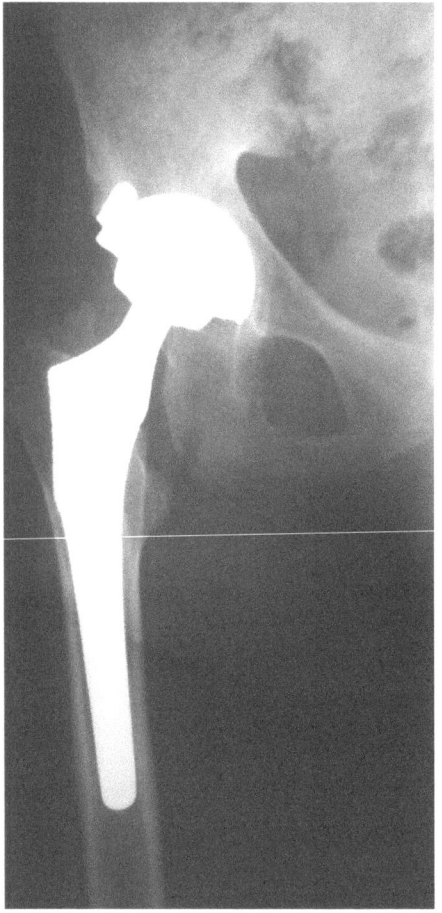

Fig. 7.18 Radiograph 1 year after primary cementless THR (PCA)

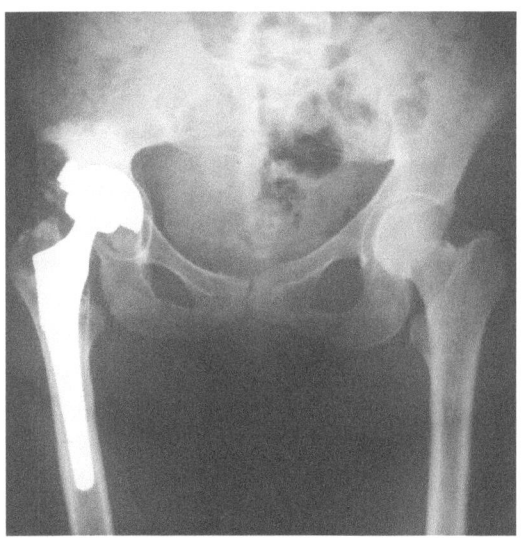

Fig. 7.19 Radiograph that was taken 10 years postoperatively

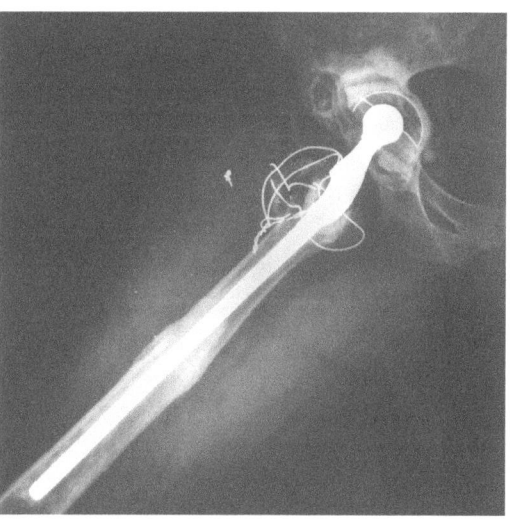

Fig. 7.21 Lateral radiograph taken 10 years after revision. Note the secure, secondary callus of the intraoperative periprosthetic fracture

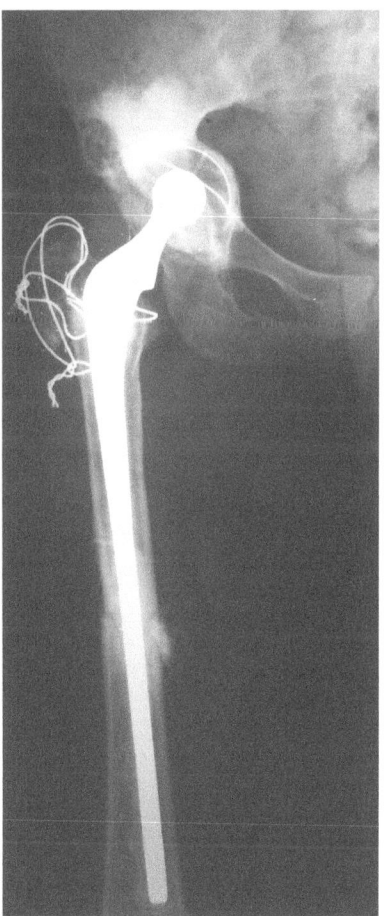

Fig. 7.20 Four months after revision and the intraoperative femoral fracture, the patient was still walking with crutches. Full weight bearing was allowed 2 months later

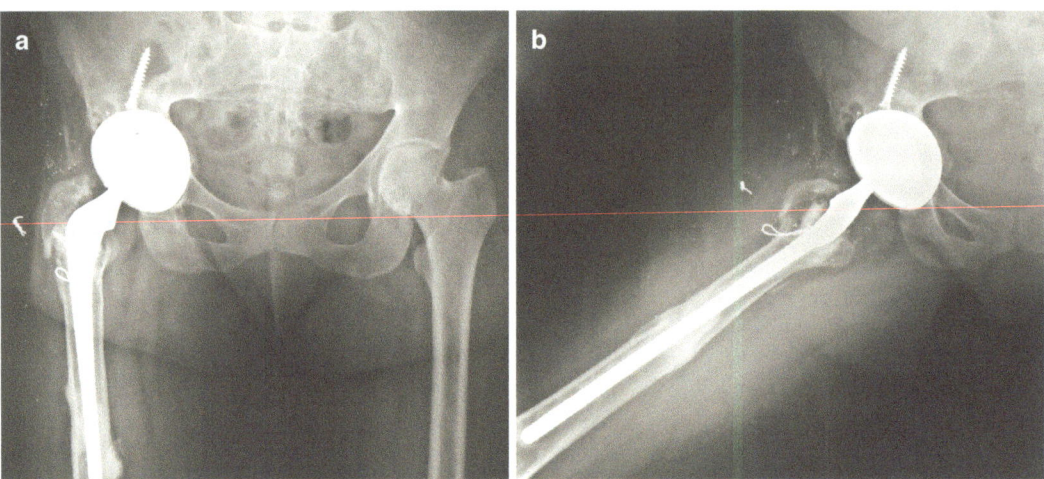

Fig. 7.22 Radiographs of (**a**) the pelvis and (**b**) the right hip taken at the last follow-up examination, 7 years after the second revision of the acetabular component and 17 years after revision of both components

THR has been considered as the operation of the century. It gives better life and hope to millions of patients with severely damaged hip joints. However, it is a demanding and irreversible operation and should be performed by experienced surgeons in specialised units and only when it is an absolute indication. Orthopaedic surgeons should protect this operation from overuse. Furthermore, they should inform the patients that it is a procedure in which the destroyed joint is removed and replaced by an artificial one. This is the reason why the term "arthroplasty" may be misleading for both the orthopaedic surgeons and the patients, and it would be better to be replaced by the term "replacement".

THR despite its excellent results, it may involve with unexpected disappointment. In the present chapter, complicated cases of THR are present to remind the "respect" we should show to this revolutionary operation.

© Springer International Publishing AG 2017
K. Lampropoulou-Adamidou, G. Hartofilakidis, *Total Hip Replacement*,
DOI 10.1007/978-3-319-53360-5_8

8.1   Case 1

This female patient was born in 1935. Pain in the right hip started at the age of 20 years. We first examined her, in 1963, when she was 28 years old. The diagnosis was OA of uncertain origin. We performed a Nissen proximal femoral osteotomy (osteotomy without displacement) combined with the Voss operation (soft tissue release). Two years later, the fixation plate was removed. At the age of 41 years, in 1976, a right LFA was needed. Seven years later, in 1983, revision of both components was performed due to aseptic loosening, and, in 2007, a re-revision of both components was also needed for the same reason. One year after the second revision, periprosthetic infection was diagnosed and removal of implants, antibiotic spacer insertion and exchange with the permanent prostheses within 6 months were performed. In 2015, 6 years later, fracture of the stem occurred and she had both components' revision in another institution.

Around the age of 47 years, she started having pain in the left hip. The diagnosis in this hip was eccentric idiopathic OA. In 1987, at the age of 52 years, she underwent a ceramic uncemented THR. Fourteen years later, in 2001, acetabular component revision was needed due to aseptic loosening. After 4 more years, the femoral component fractured, but the patient refused the recommended operation. Revision of both components of this hip was performed 6 years later, in 2011, 24 years after primary replacement.

At the latest follow-up, the patient was 81 years old and had nine operations in the right hip and three in the left. She had painless hips with indoor activities (Figs. 8.1–8.14).

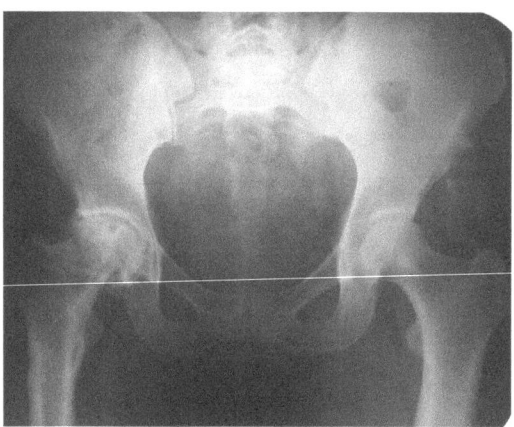

Fig. 8.2   This radiograph was taken 4 years after the previous operation. The patient had temporary clinical and radiographic improvement. The left hip at that time was normal

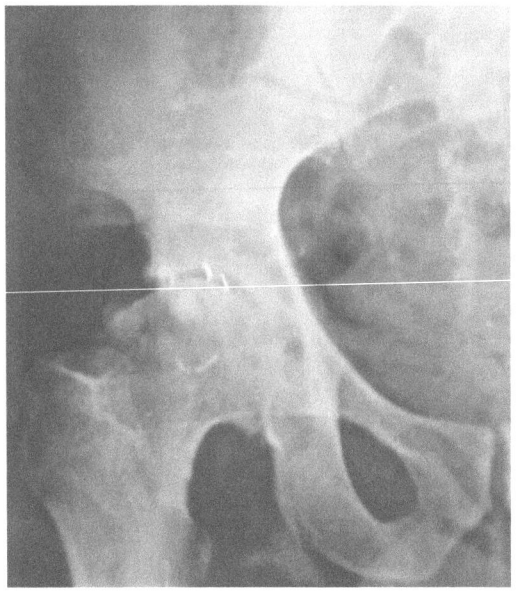

Fig. 8.1   Radiograph of the right hip made in 1963, when the patient was 28 years old and first visited us. We diagnosed OA the origin of which could not be defined. A Nissen subtrochanteric osteotomy combined with the Voss operation was performed

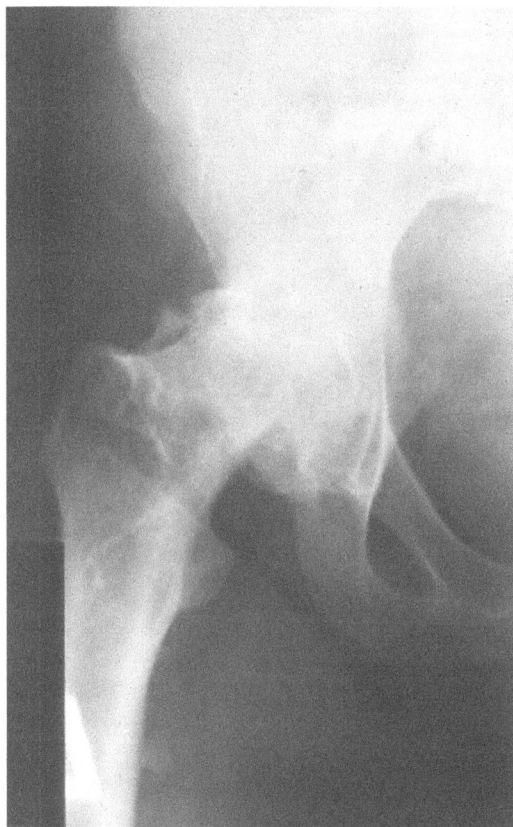

Fig. 8.3 In 1976, at the age of 42 years, she had a severe deterioration and a right LFA was decided

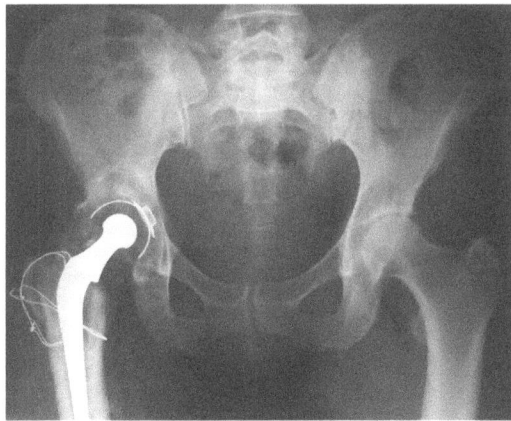

Fig. 8.4 Radiograph after LFA of the right hip. The left hip was normal. The patient remained symptoms-free for the next 6 years

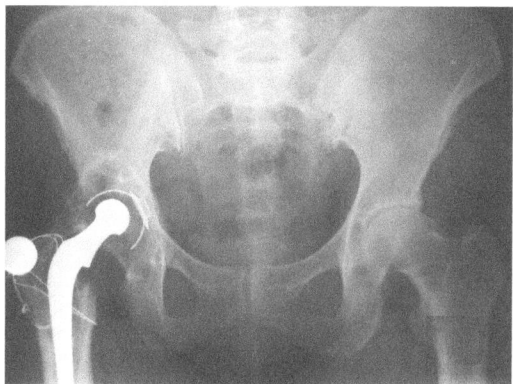

Fig. 8.5 Radiograph made 7 years after LFA of the right hip. Wear of the acetabulum and implants' loosening in consideration of patient's symptoms led to the decision of both components' revision. The onset of eccentric OA of the left hip was noticed

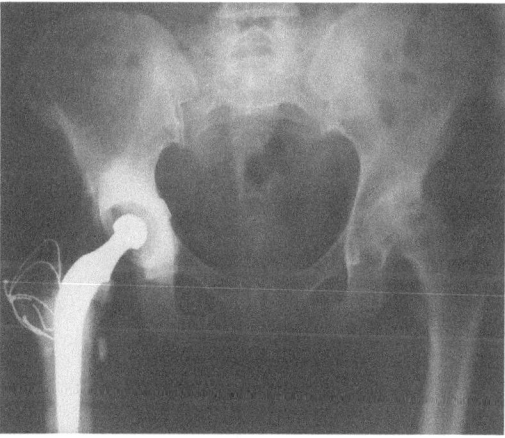

Fig. 8.6 Three years after revision of the right hip. The left hip rapidly worsened

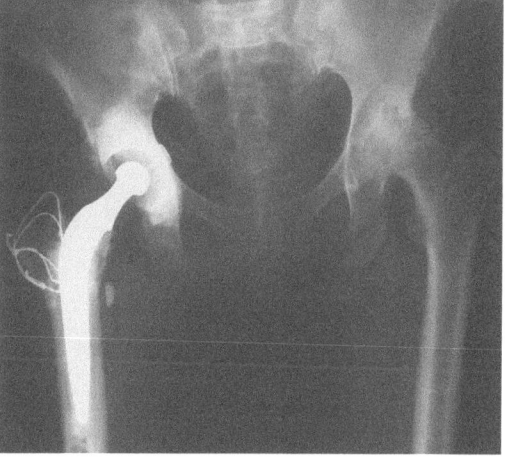

Fig. 8.7 After one more year, when the left THR was decided in 1987

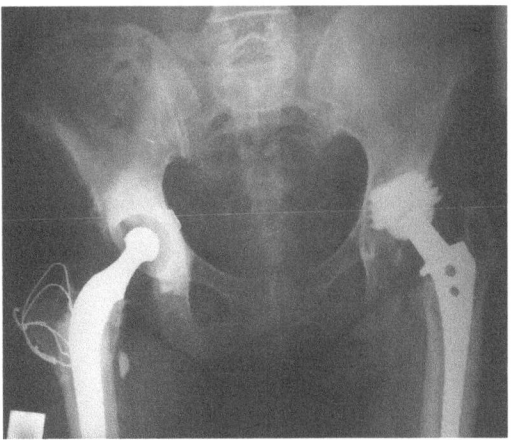

Fig. 8.8 One year after ceramic uncemented THR of the left hip and 5 years after revision of the right. The patient remained free of symptoms in both hips

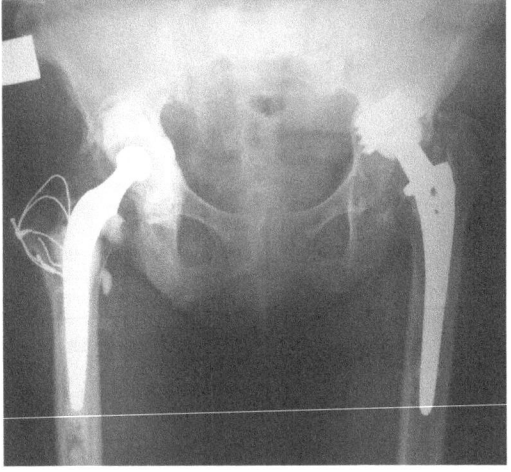

Fig. 8.9 Radiograph taken in 2001, 18 years after revision of the right hip and 14 years after primary replacement of the left. There is aseptic loosening of the left cup, which was subsequently revised

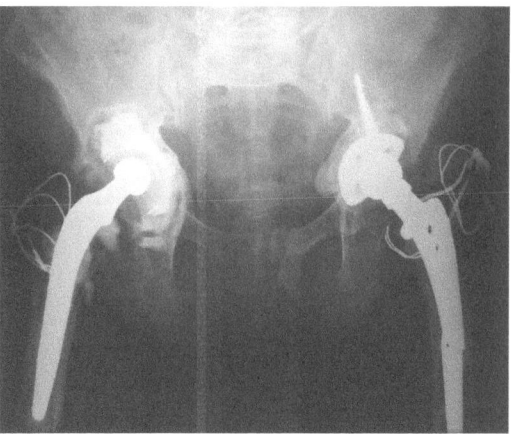

Fig. 8.10 Radiograph taken in 2005, 22 years after revision of the right hip and 4 years after revision of the left cup when fracture of the ceramic left stem occurred. At the same time, implant loosening of the right hip was also noticed. Two years later, re-revision of the right THR was followed. The patient refused a reoperation of the left hip

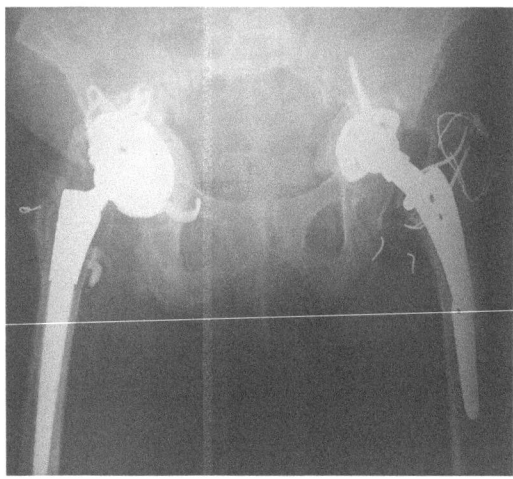

Fig. 8.11 Radiograph after both component re-revision of the right THR. One year later, removal of implants, antibiotic spacer insertion and exchange with the permanent prostheses within 6 months were performed because of periprosthetic joint infection. After 2 more years, in 2009, she had a revision of the left hip

Fig. 8.12 In 2015, fracture of the right stem occurred and another revision of both components was followed in another institution

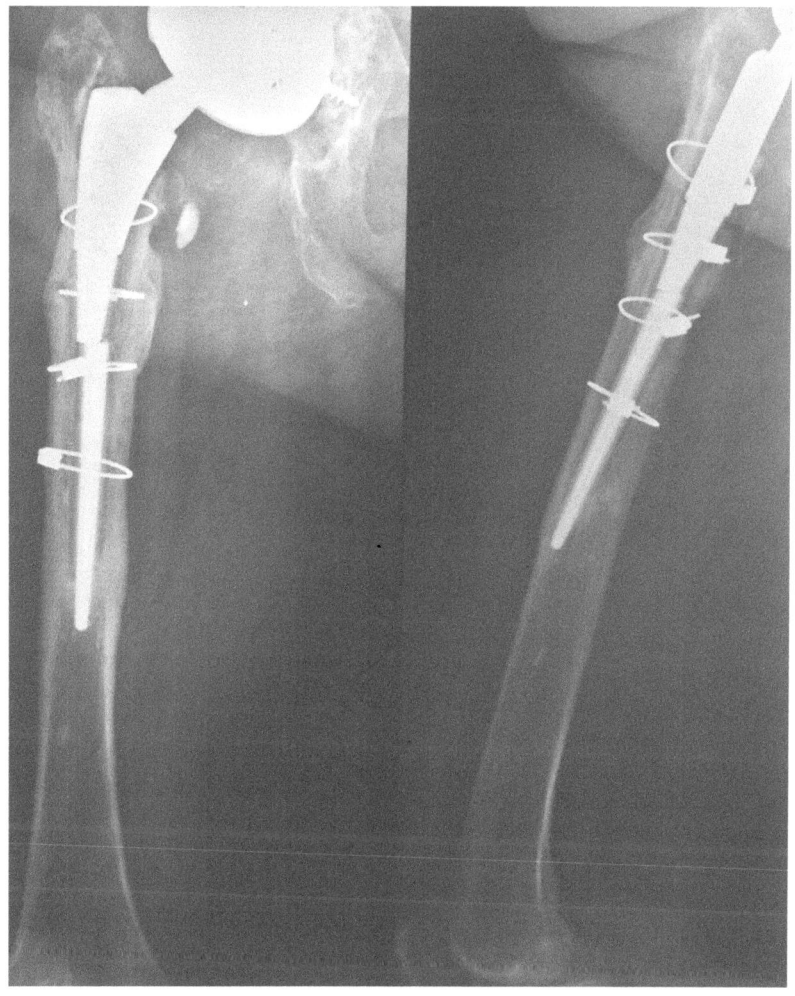

Fig. 8.13 Picture of the right broken stem

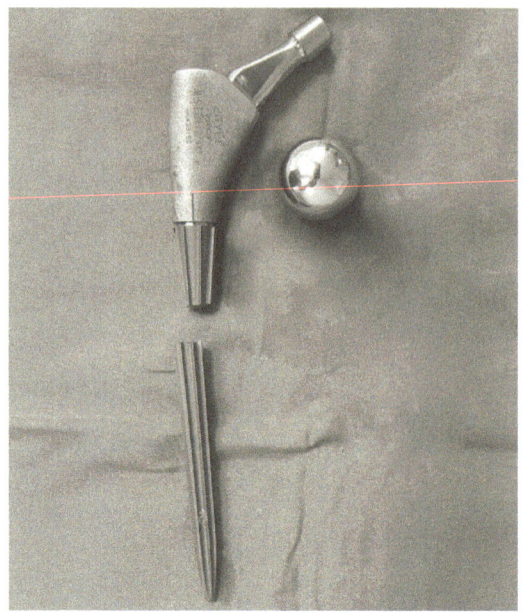

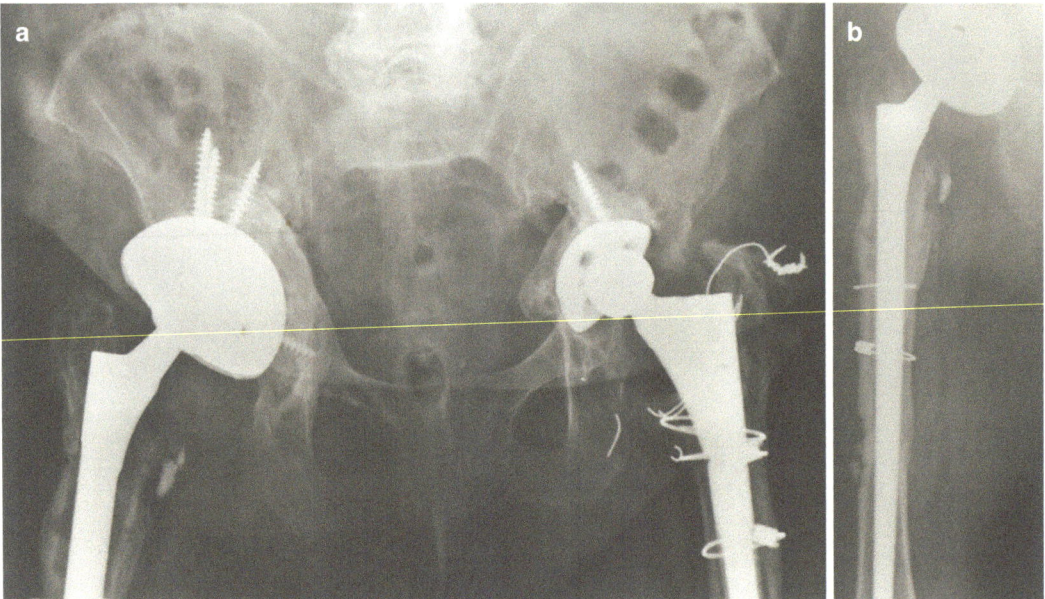

Fig. 8.14 The latest follow-up radiograph of (**a**) the pelvis and (**b**) the right hip that was taken, in 2016, after the last revision of the right hip. The adventure of this patient started before 53 years

8.2   Case 2

This female patient was born in 1923. At the age of 54 years, she began to have pain in the left hip because of eccentric idiopathic OA. Four years later, in 1981, she had a THR in another institution, which was revised by the same surgeon after 5 years.

In 1989, 3 years after revision, we first examined her, and we recognised that a second revision was needed because of aseptic loosening of both components. A series of operations was followed:

- One year after the second revision, in 1990, a periprosthetic fracture of the femur just distal to the cement mantle of the stem occurred and was treated with open reduction and internal fixation, as the stem was considered stable.
- In 1995, a second periprosthetic fracture occurred just proximally to the previous

healed fracture, and another surgeon at that time decided to treat it with a third revision.
- Eight years later, in 2003, a fourth revision was followed because of aseptic loosening of both components.
- After one more year, at the age of 81 years, she underwent cementless THR of the right hip which was diagnosed as having idiopathic OA.
- In 2005, dislocation of the left hip occurred because of loosening and migration of the components. Her surgeon suggested another operation and the patient refused.

The patient returned to us for consultation, in 2009, 5 years after the latter operation. Loosening and migration of both components of the left hip was noticed. The patient refused any further intervention. She had already six operations on the left hip and one on the right. We recently contracted her by phone. She was 93 years old and had limited indoor activities with the use of a walker (Figs. 8.15–8.23).

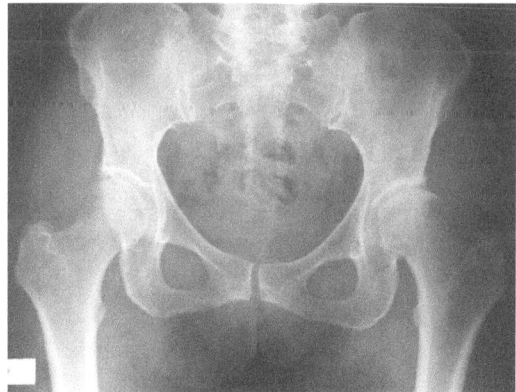

Fig. 8.15 This radiograph was taken, in 1977, when the patient was 54 years old and started having pain in the left hip because of eccentric idiopathic OA

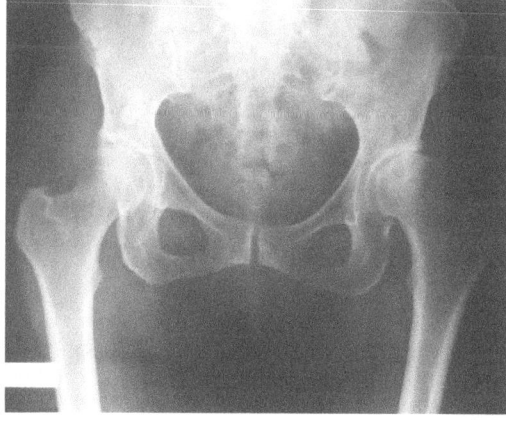

Fig. 8.16 Radiograph taken before primary THR performed in another institution, in 1981

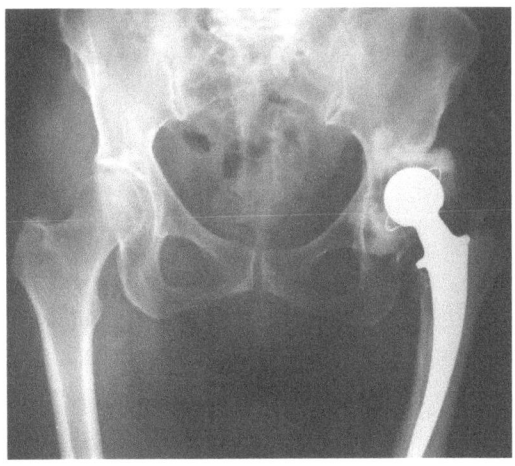

Fig. 8.17 Four years after primary THR. Revision was performed 1 year later in 1986

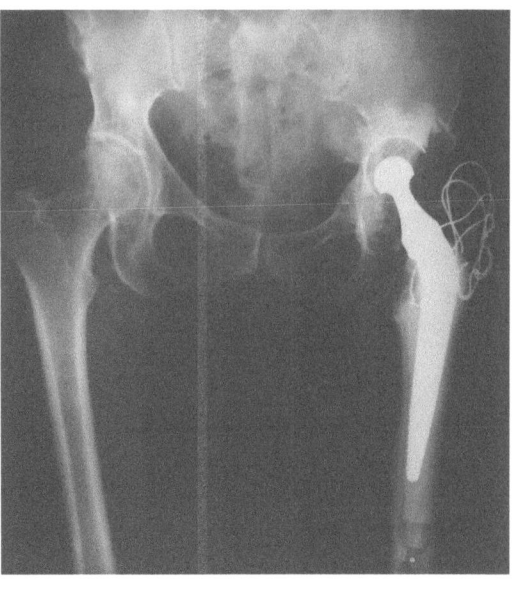

Fig. 8.19 After the second revision. Note that the stem did not bypass the cortical defect

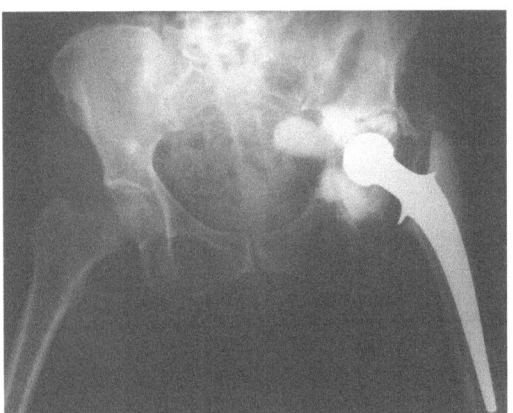

Fig. 8.18 Radiograph when the patient first visited us in 1989. Both components were definitely loose

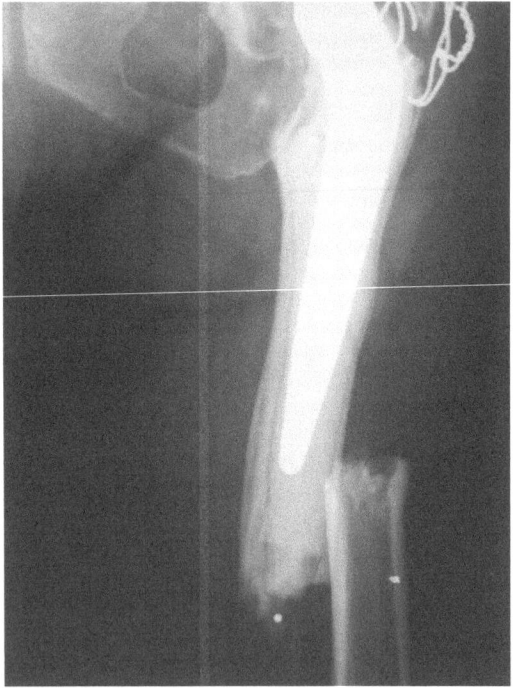

Fig. 8.20 One year later, a transverse periprosthetic fracture occurred just distal to the cement mantle of the stem, treated with osteosynthesis

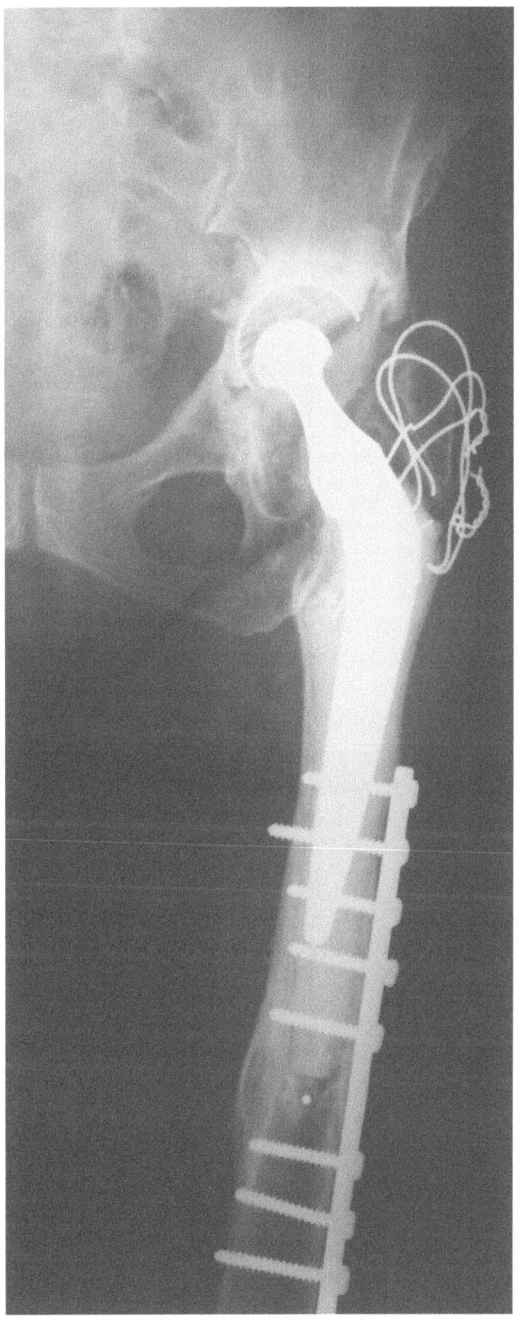

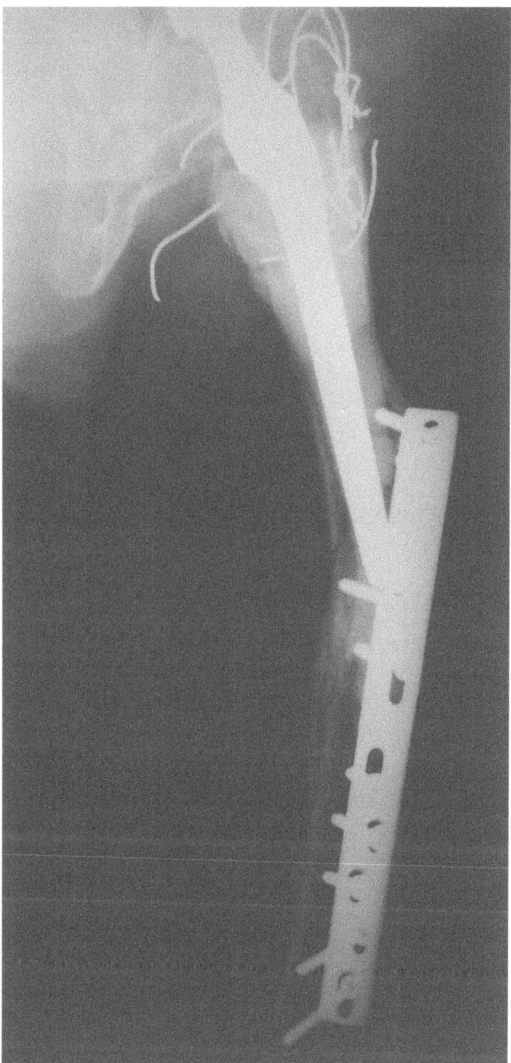

Fig. 8.22 A second periprosthetic fracture occurred just proximally to the previous healed fracture, in 1995, treated by a third surgeon with one more revision. Eight years later, in 2003, a fourth revision was performed because of the aseptic loosening of the components by the same surgeon. In 2004, she underwent a THR of the right hip. In 2005, dislocation of the left hip occurred and her surgeon suggested a new operation. The patient refused any further intervention

Fig. 8.21 Four years after osteosynthesis, in 1994, there is a complete union of the fracture

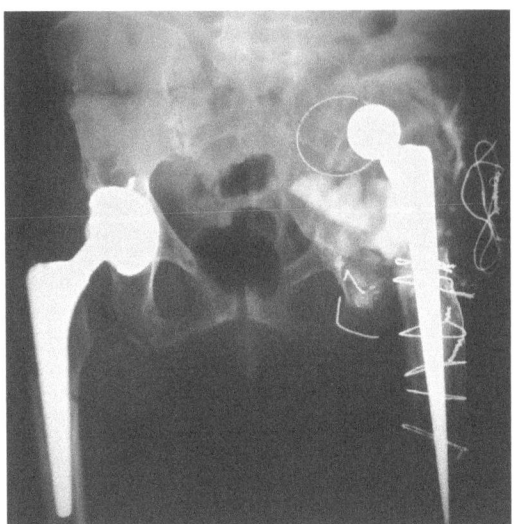

Fig. 8.23 The latest radiograph, when the patient returned to us for consultation, in 2009. She was 86 years old and had definitely loose components of the left dislocated THR. The bad general condition and the advanced age of the patient did not permit any further intervention. Palliative treatment was recommended

8.3 Case 3

This female patient was born in 1941 with CHD of both hips. She had no treatment in infancy and was limping since then. She started to have pain around the age of 25 years particularly in the right hip. The patient was referred to us in 1981, at the age of 40 years. She had high dislocation of the left hip and low dislocation of the right. She was treated with LFA in both hips within 5 months. Eight years later, in 1989, the left hip was revised because of aseptic loosening.

Since then, she had, in 1996, a second revision of the left femoral component because of peri-prosthetic femoral fracture. In 1999, 18 years after primary right LFA, revision of both components because of aseptic loosening was performed. In 2011, a second revision of the left cup was considered necessary also because of aseptic loosening. In 2014, aseptic loosening of both components of the right THR led to a second revision of this hip.

Totally, the patient had four operations on the left hip and three on the right. She was contacted recently by phone. She was 75 years old, and she had limited indoor activities, walking with the use of a walker without hip pain. She stated: "All I want is a life without pain. I have faith in God and my surgeons and I believe that everything will go well" (Figs. 8.24–8.31).

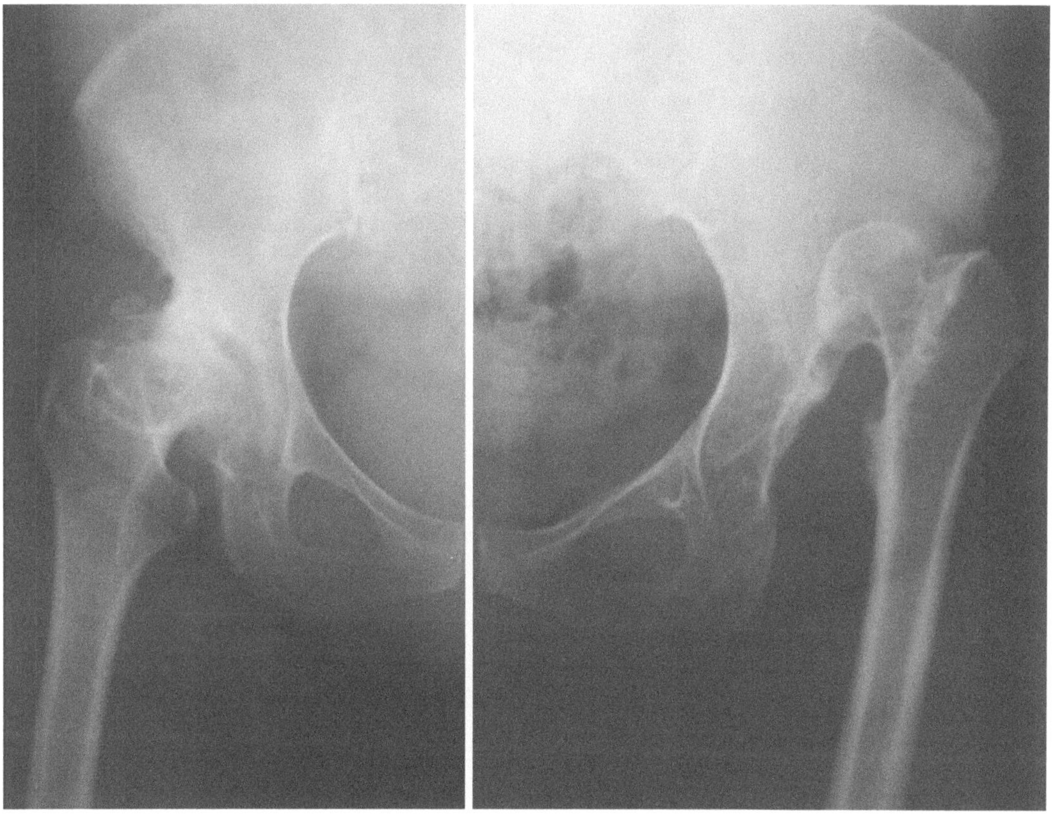

Fig. 8.24 Preoperative radiograph, when the patient was 40 years old and was diagnosed as having high dislocation of the left hip and low dislocation of the right

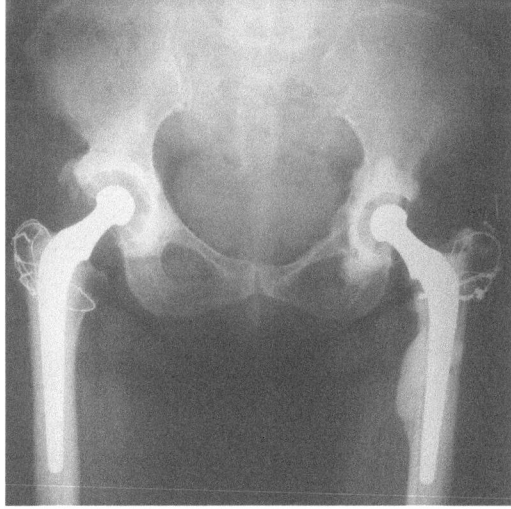

Fig. 8.25 Six years after primary replacements. Note that cement had escaped from the medial cortex of the left femur

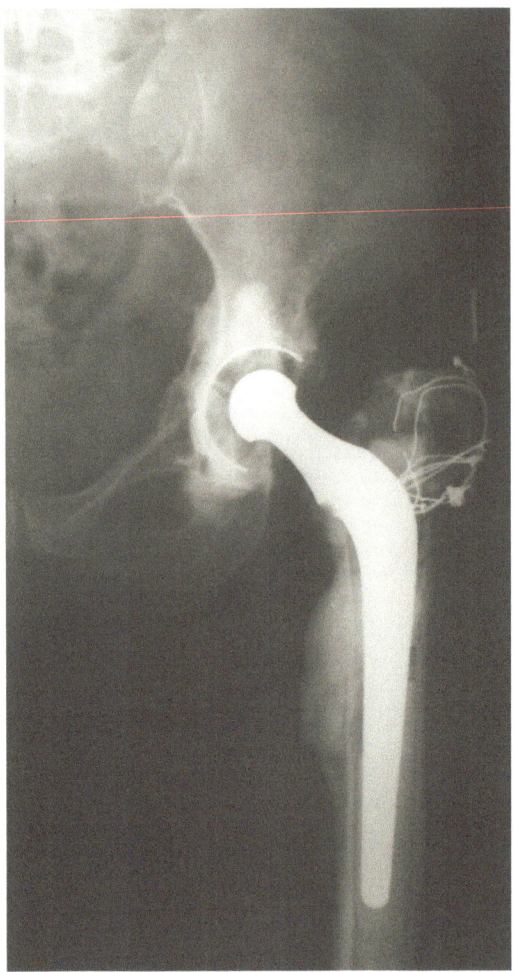

Fig. 8.26 Pre-revision of the left hip, 8 years after primary THR

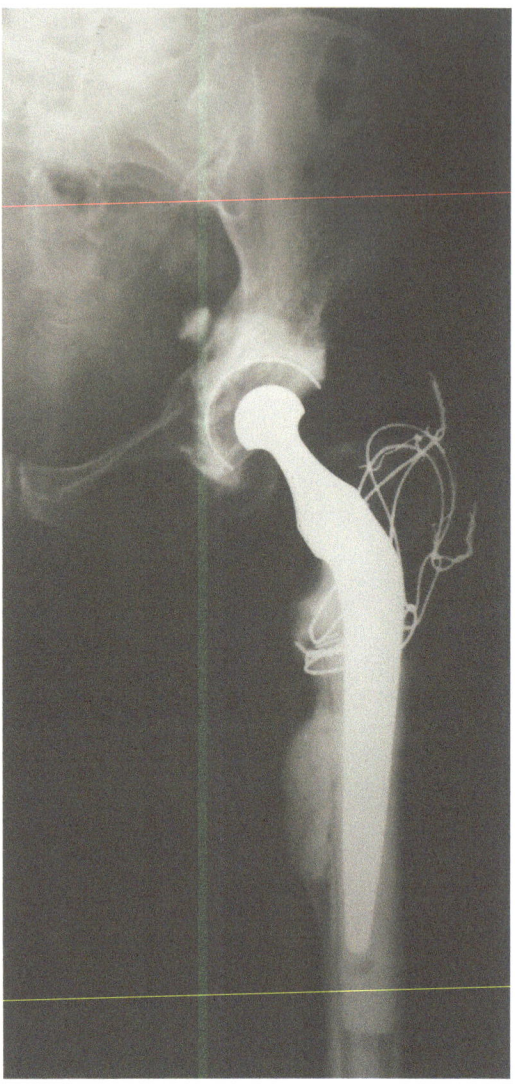

Fig. 8.27 Radiograph after revision of the left hip

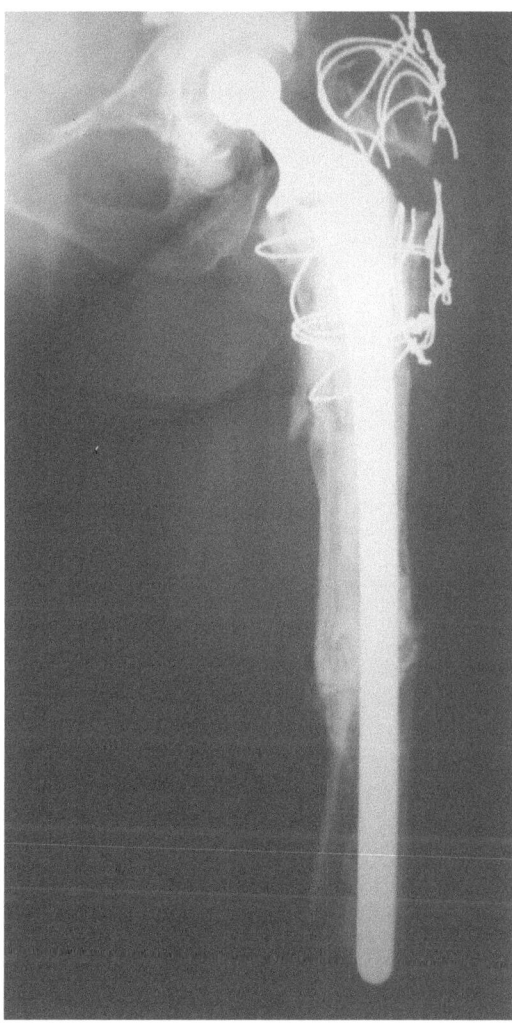

Fig. 8.28 In 1996, 7 years after the previous revision of the left stem, re-revision was performed because of periprosthetic fracture

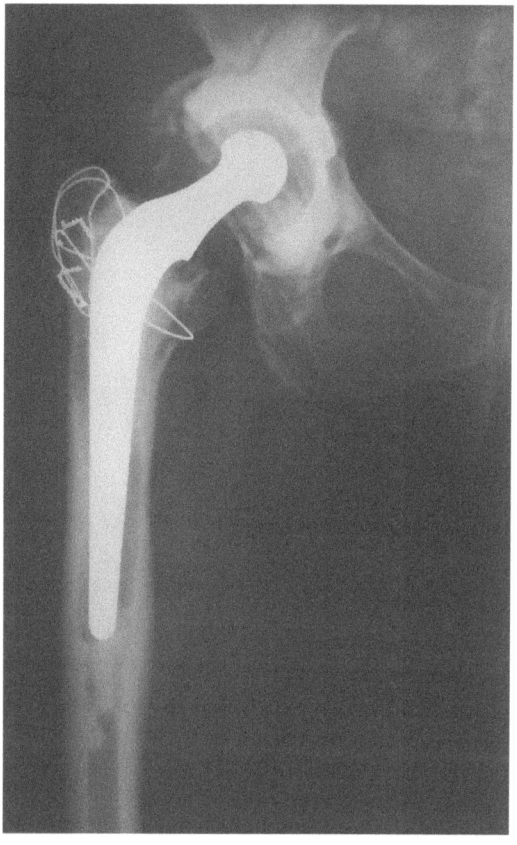

Fig. 8.29 Radiograph taken in 1999, 18 years after primary LFAs, both components' aseptic loosening of the right hip led to a revision. Two years later, a second revision of the left cup was considered necessary also because of aseptic loosening

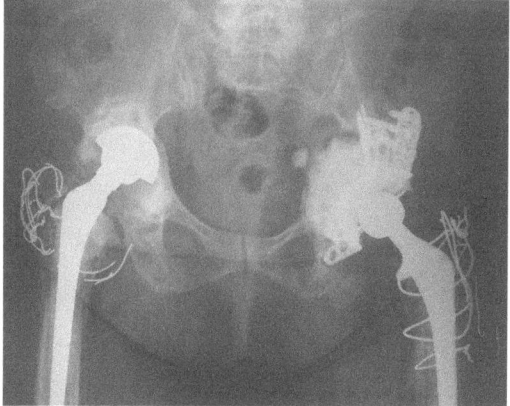

Fig. 8.30 Radiograph taken in 2012, 1 year after revision of the left cup and 3 years after revision of the right THR. After two more years, aseptic loosening of both components of the right THR led to a second revision of this hip

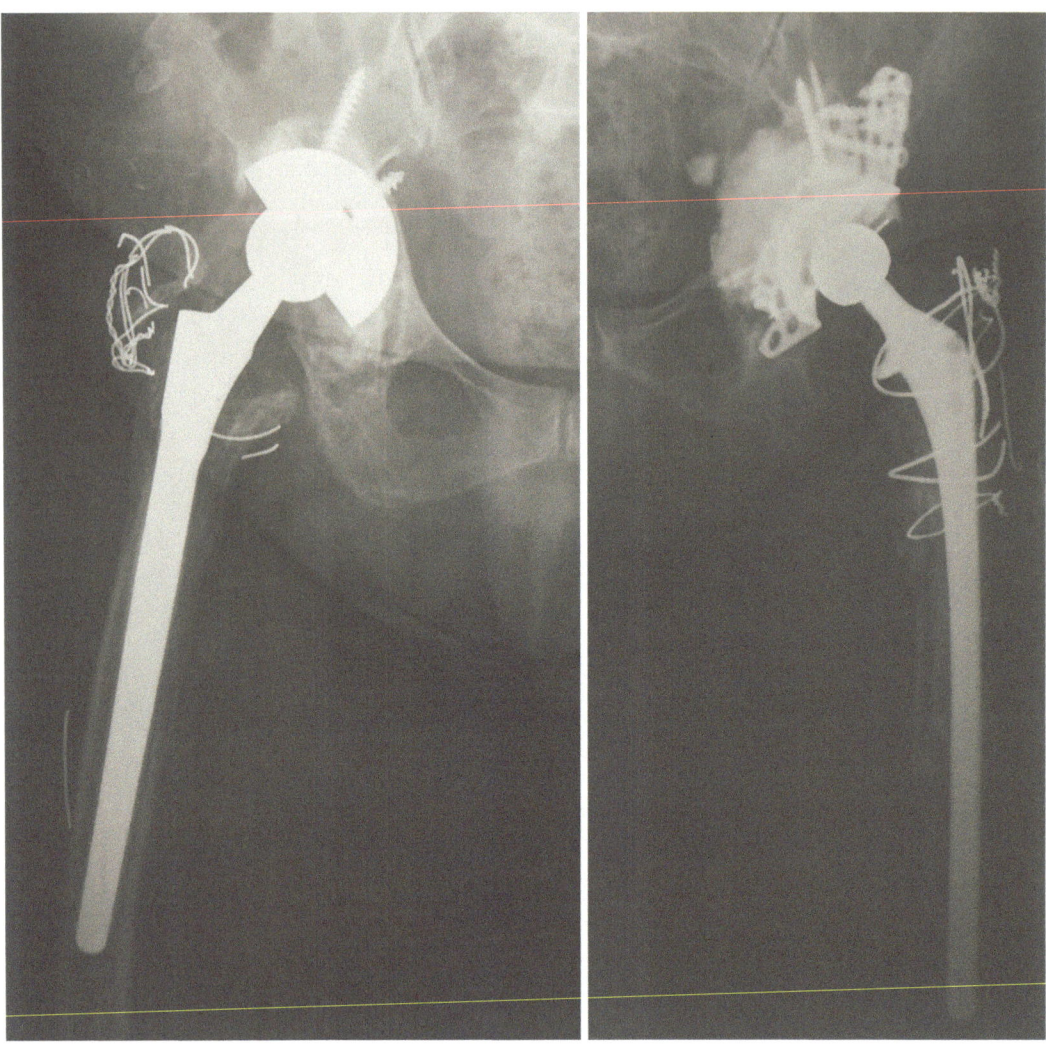

Fig. 8.31 The last follow-up radiographs, when the patient was 75 years old, 2 years after the re-revision of the right hip

8.4   Case 4

This female patient was born in 1935 with CHD of both hips. She was limping since infancy. At the age of 23 years, her physician treated her with Schanz subtrochanteric osteotomy of both hips. She continued to limp, and around the age of 35 years, she started having pain in both hips. She was referred to us in 1990, at the age of 55 years, with high dislocation of both hips. She had severe pain, heavy limping and great deformity of the pelvis. She had difficulty walking, even with the use of crutches.

We performed LFAs of the left and right hip within 3 weeks. One year later, the left stem was revised due to early loosening. For the next 14 years, she was walking with the use of a crutch, and she only had occasional pain in both hips.

Nonetheless, from 2005, she was worsening and underwent five more operations:

- In 2005, she underwent revision of the right hip and re-revision of the left stem, because of aseptic loosening.
- Three years later, she sustained a right peri-prosthetic femoral fracture that was treated with internal osteosynthesis.
- One year after osteosynthesis, fracture of the fixation plate occurred and re-revision of the right hip was performed.
- In 2011, the left cup was revised because of loosening complicated by peroneal nerve palsy and acute periprosthetic joint infection treated with surgical debridement.

Totally, she had 5 operations on the left and 4 on the right hip. We examined the patient at the age of 80 years, in 2015. She had slight hip pain and was walking with two crutches (Figs. 8.32–8.39).

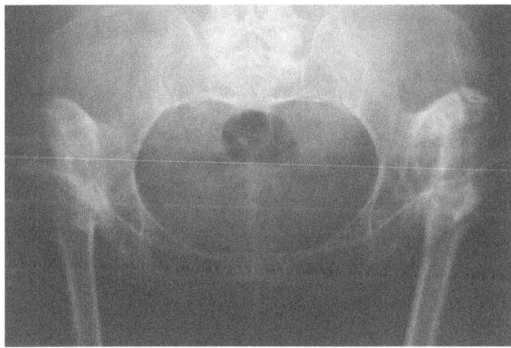

Fig. 8.32 Radiograph taken in 1990 prior to LFAs when the patient was 55 years old

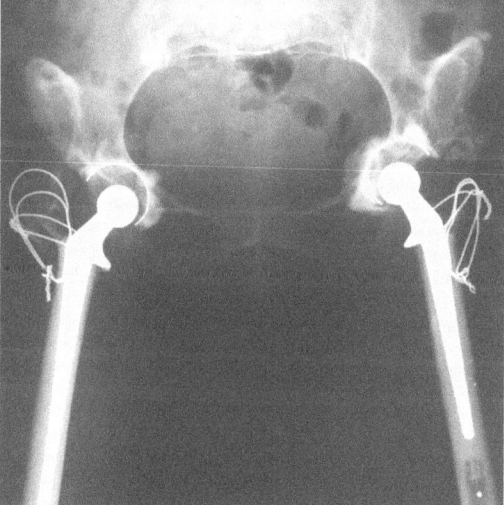

Fig. 8.33 One year after primary replacements. Revision of the left stem was followed due to early loosening

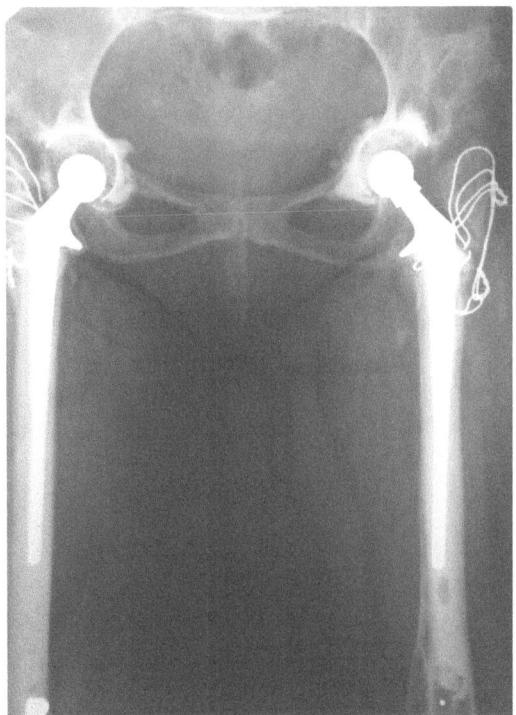

Fig. 8.34 Two months after revision of the left stem

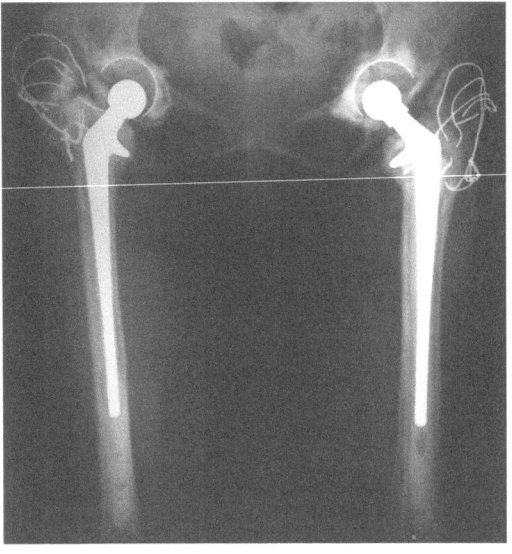

Fig. 8.35 In 2003, 12 years after primary replacement of the right hip and 11 years after revision of the left stem. During the next 2 years, osteolysis around both stems was increasing, followed by revision of both components of the right hip and re-revision of the left stem

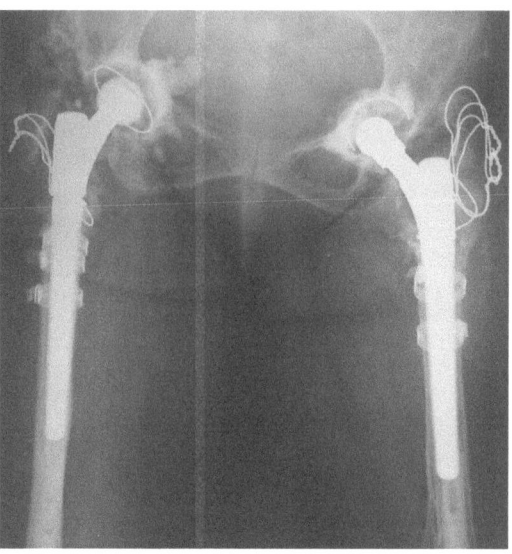

Fig. 8.36 Radiograph after revision of both components of the right hip and re-revision of the left stem

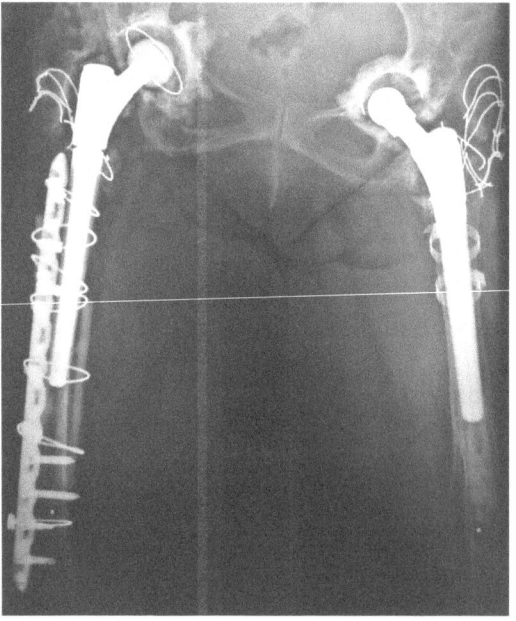

Fig. 8.37 Radiograph taken in 2008 after right peri-prosthetic fracture that was treated with internal osteosynthesis

Fig. 8.38 Failure of the fixation plate of the right femur led to another revision with a special stem in 2009. Two years later, revision of the left acetabular component because of aseptic loosening was also needed

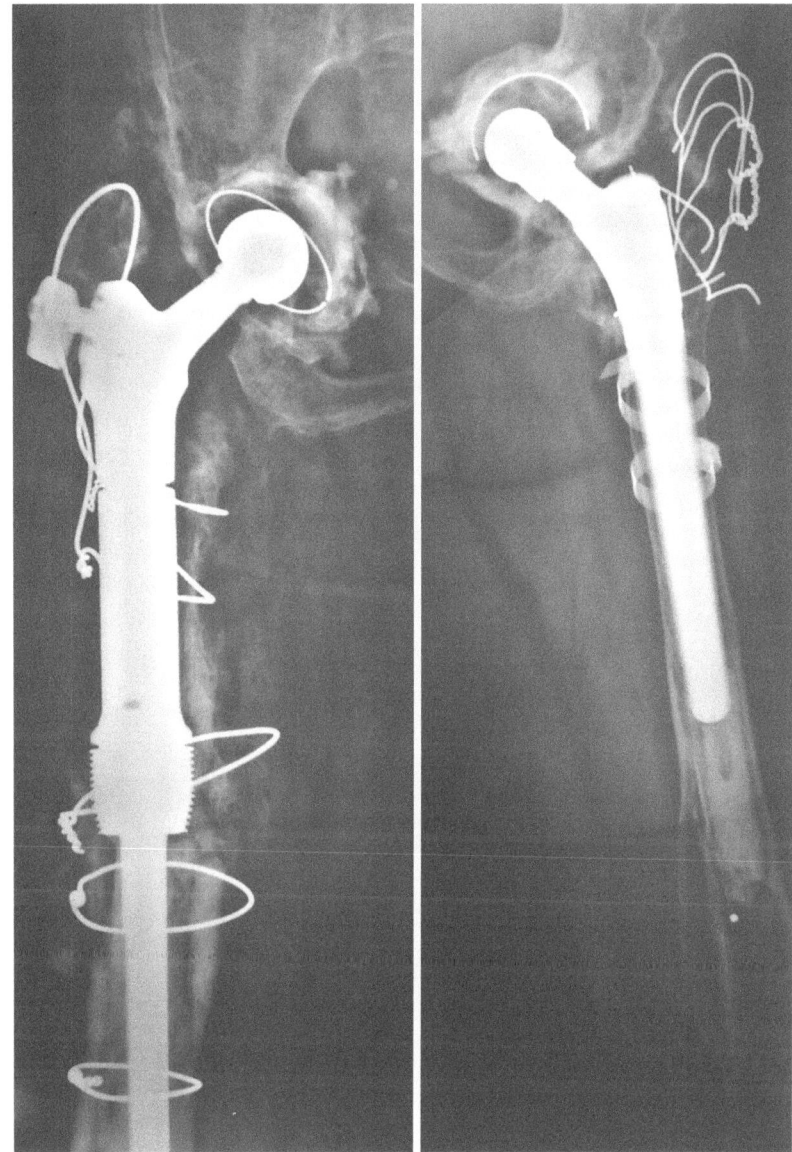

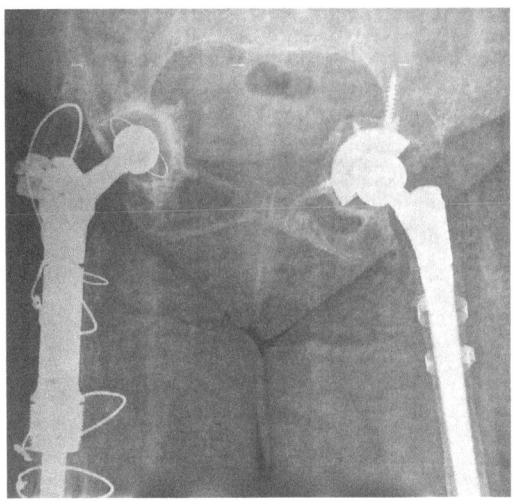

Fig. 8.39 The most recent radiograph was taken 24 years after the first patient's operation

8.5   Case 5

This female patient was born in 1949. At the age of 33 years, in 1982, she had a THR of her left dysplastic hip in a peripheral hospital. In the following years, she had no constant follow-up. Eight years later, in 1990, she was admitted to our department with extended destruction of the upper femur and the acetabulum. Revision of both components with cotyloplasty was performed. Since then, she underwent the following three operations on the left hip. Femoral and acetabular components because of aseptic loosening were re-revised, 3 and 4 years after previous revision, respectively. A third revision of the stem was followed in 2002, when the patient was 53 years old.

In addition, she had right TKR, at the age of 53 years, and right THR, 10 years later in 2012. At the last follow-up, at the age of 66 years, despite the numerous previous operations, she had pain-free hips and knees, no limping and satisfactory activity level (Figs. 8.40–8.51).

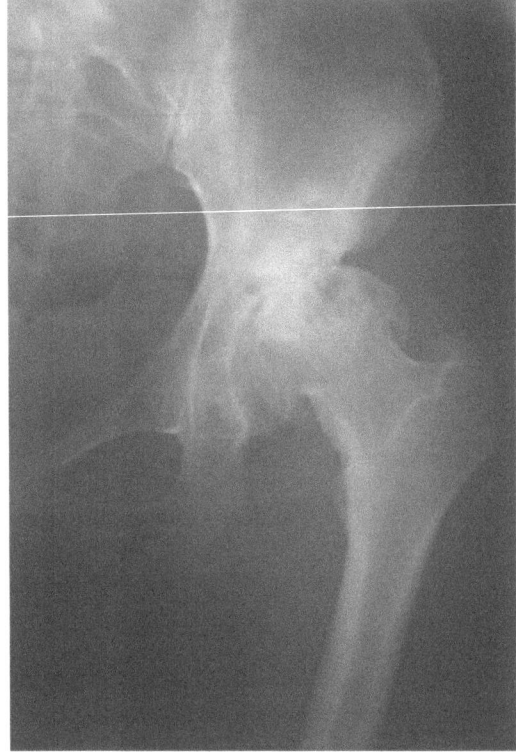

Fig. 8.40 This radiograph was taken when the patient was 33 years old, in 1982. She had secondary OA of the left hip because of dysplasia. THR was performed in another institution

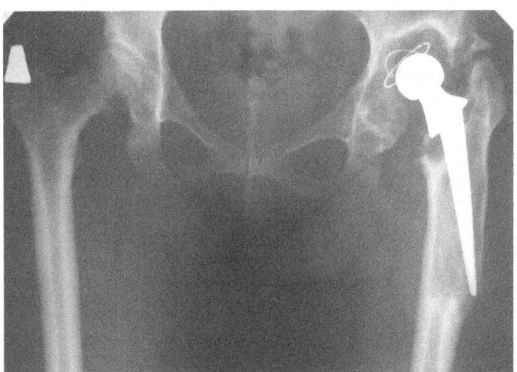

Fig. 8.41 Radiograph taken when we examined the patient, 7 years postoperatively in 1989. She had no constant follow-up after primary THR. Note that the neck-shaft angle of the asymptomatic right hip was varus (110°) and the acetabulum retroverted

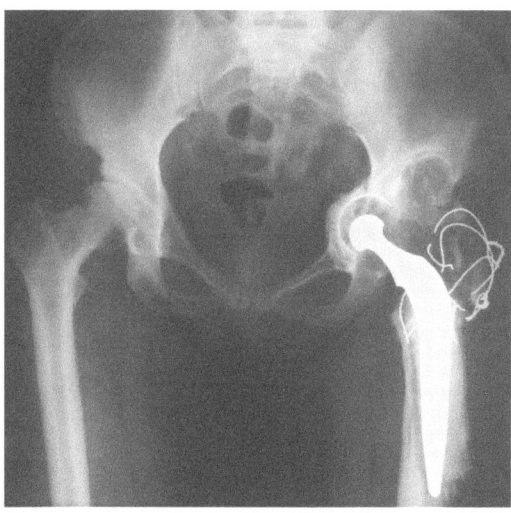

Fig. 8.43 Three years after revision, in 1993, a re-revision of the stem was needed

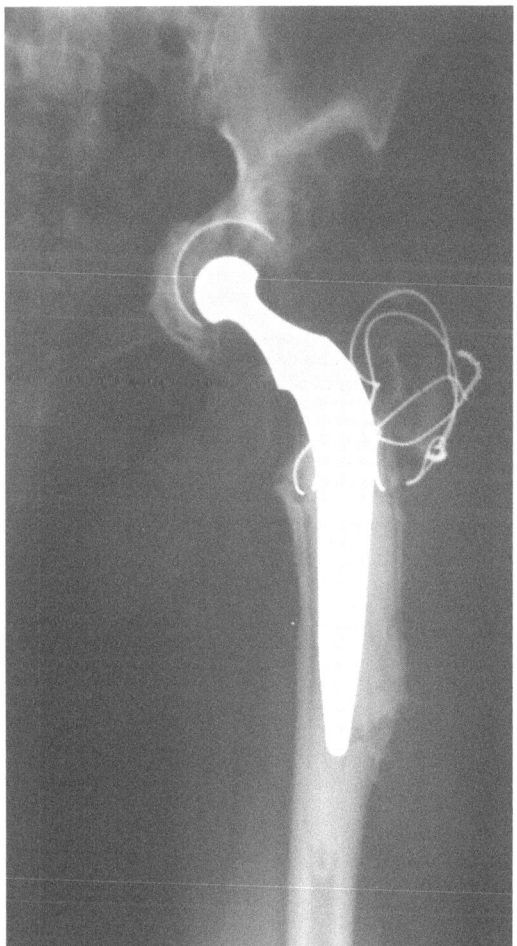

Fig. 8.42 One year after revision of both components with cotyloplasty. Of note, the stem had not bypassed the femoral shaft defect

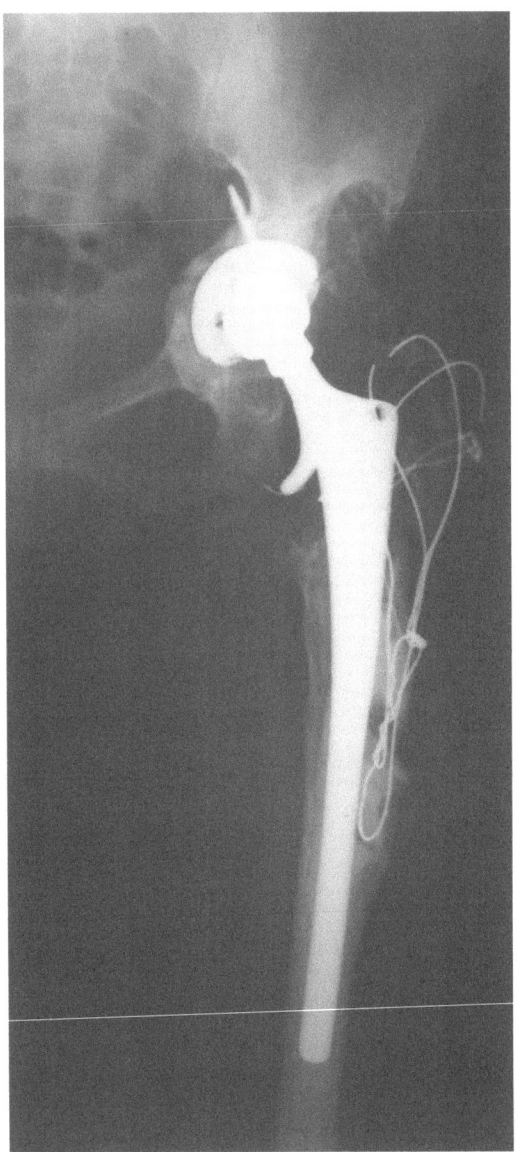 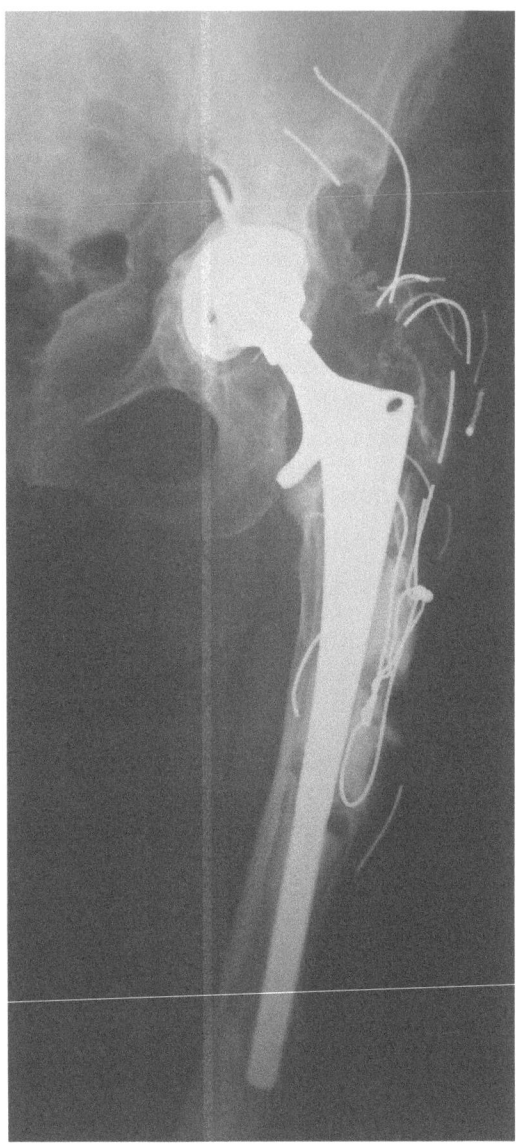

Fig. 8.44 One year later, a re-revision of the acetabular component was considered necessary

Fig. 8.45 The stem failed again, 9 years after its re-revision, and was revised in 2002 for third time with the use of more complicated techniques

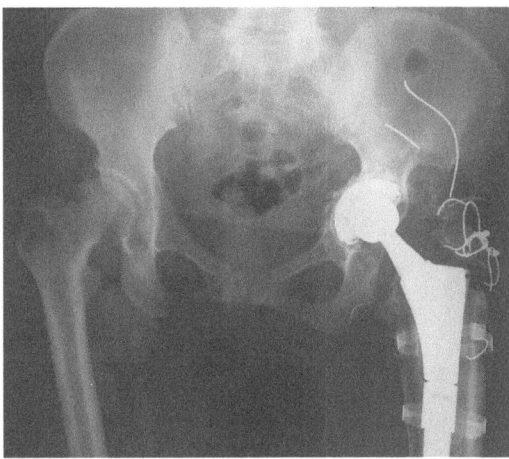

Fig. 8.46 One year after the latter operation, the right hip remained asymptomatic although degenerative changes had been initiated

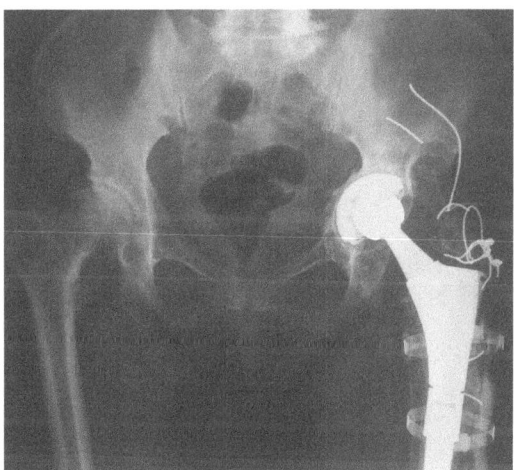

Fig. 8.47 This radiograph was taken 10 years after the third revision of the left stem in 2012. Right hip pain and limping started 1 year previously, when the patient was 62 years old, followed by right cementless THR. Twenty-three years after we first had recognised the morphologic variations of that hip, it is ambiguous if the osteoarthritic development was due to morphologic variations of the joint or to idiopathic OA

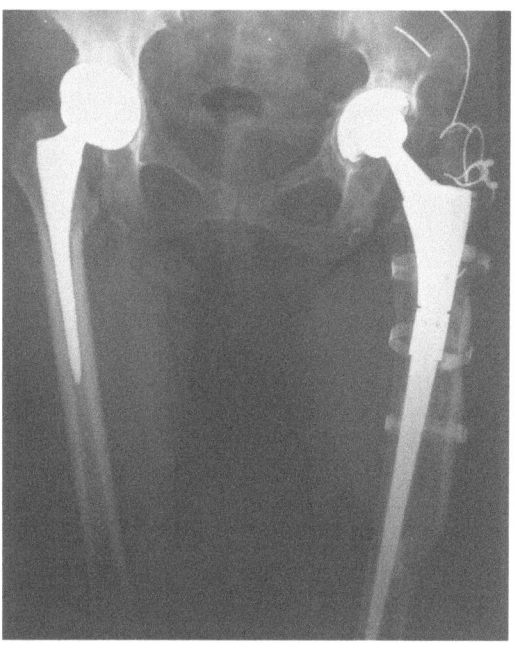

Fig. 8.48 Three years after THR of the right hip and 33 years after the primary left THR

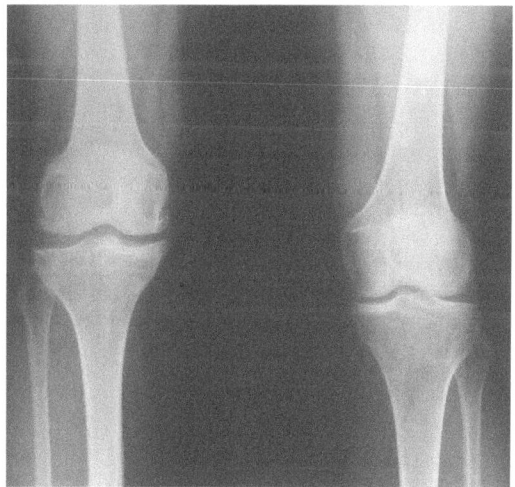

Fig. 8.49 Anteroposterior radiograph of both knees, when the patient was 45 years old. She had a vague pain in the right knee

Fig. 8.50 Deterioration of OA of the right knee within 8 years

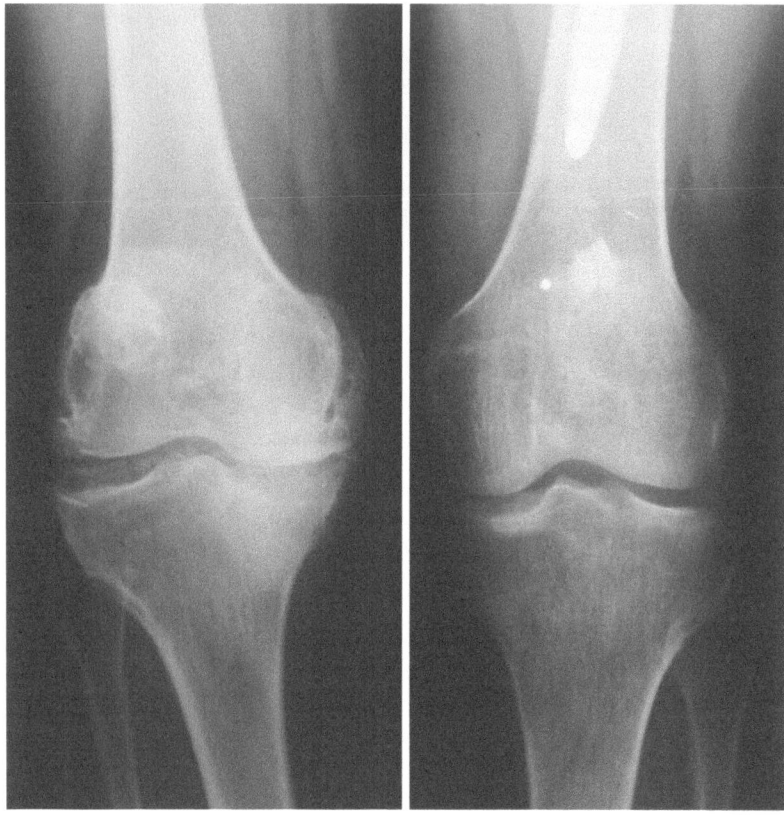

Fig. 8.51 Thirteen years after right TKR

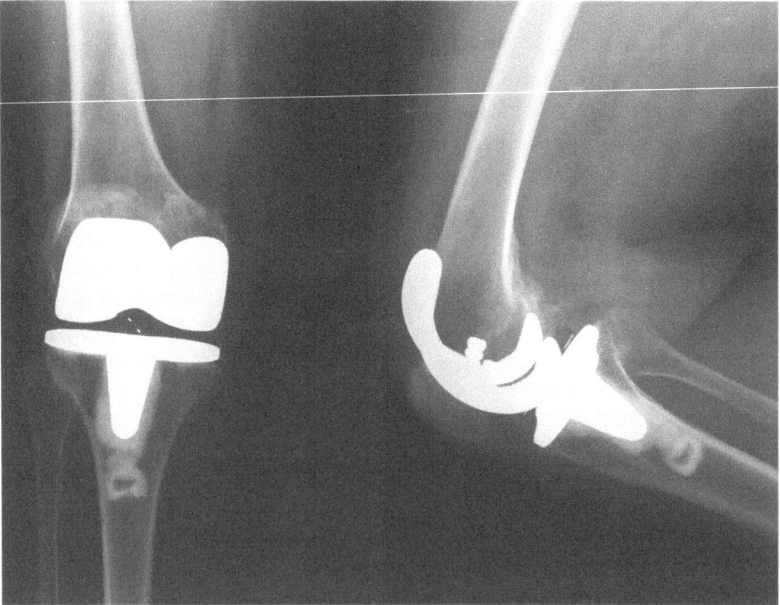

Miscellaneous

This chapter includes miscellaneous selected cases of interest.

- Case 1 presents the revascularisation of a frozen femoral head allograft used to replace the destroyed bearing surface of the acetabulum after a failed Thompson endoprosthesis.
- In case 2, the long-term delay of revision after periprosthetic osteolysis caused by severe wear of an all-polyethylene Charnley cup is presented.
- Case 3 is an example of severe complications following THR of a hip with high dislocation performed without trochanteric osteotomy.
- The successful outcome of removal of a Brooker grade 4 heterotopic ossification causing complete ankylosis of the hip performed 20 years after primary replacement is presented in case 4.
- In case 5, the uncomplicated result of a THR followed for 28 years that was performed in a patient with chronic osteomyelitis in the contralateral tibia is presented.
- Case 6 is an example of slow development of secondary OA of a hip with low dislocation, needed THR 25 years after the onset of

symptoms, and rapid deterioration of the contralateral hip with eccentric idiopathic OA that underwent THR 3 years after the first appearance of osteoarthritic changes.
- Cases 7, 8 and 9 present three generations of female patients from the same family with CHD treated with different methods according to the methods used at that period of time.
- Case 10 presents the long-term stability of a long stem with distal cemented fixation, performed 21 years ago, for the revision of a failed THR with complete absence of the outer cortex of the proximal femur.
- In case 11, the 30-year outcome of a cement-in-cement revision of a failed endoprosthesis with extended osteolysis of the proximal femur is presented.
- Case 12 presents the long-term outcome of a hybrid THR of both hips after the previous Chiary osteotomy was performed, according to the patient, by Chiary himself.
- Case 13 is an example of long-term outcome of hybrid THR performed in a patient with CHD of a borderline type between low and high dislocation. Definite diagnosis was secured by using 3D CT scan.

© Springer International Publishing AG 2017
K. Lampropoulou-Adamidou, G. Hartofilakidis, *Total Hip Replacement*,
DOI 10.1007/978-3-319-53360-5_9

9.1   Case 1

This male patient was born in 1928. At the age of
45 years, he sustained a right femoral neck fracture treated by his physician with Thompson
endoprosthesis. Two years postoperatively, he
started limping. In the next years, his leg was
gradually shortening and the limping was
increasing. The patient never had a follow-up
examination since his operation. He consulted
us, in 1988, at the age of 60 years, 15 years after
his surgery. He was limping heavily and was
walking with the use of crutches. He had 3 cm

shortening of the right leg. Radiographically, the
prosthesis had penetrated the roof of the acetabulum and had migrated anterosuperiorly. We performed revision with LFA using frozen femoral
head allograft fixed with screws to fill the spherical defect of the pelvis. The graft revascularised
and the prosthesis remained stable for the next
years. His last follow-up examination was performed 10 years after revision. He was 70 years
old and he had normal activity without pain or
limping on his right hip. He died 3 years later
from reason unrelated to his hip problem (Figs.
9.1–9.6).

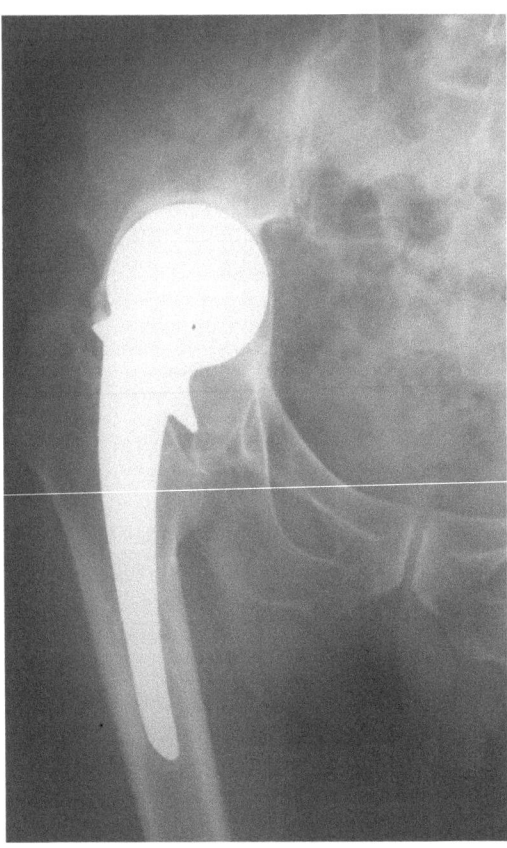

Fig. 9.1 Radiograph 15 years after implantation of
Thompson endoprosthesis, when the patient first visited
us. The prosthesis had penetrated the roof of the acetabulum and had migrated anterosuperiorly

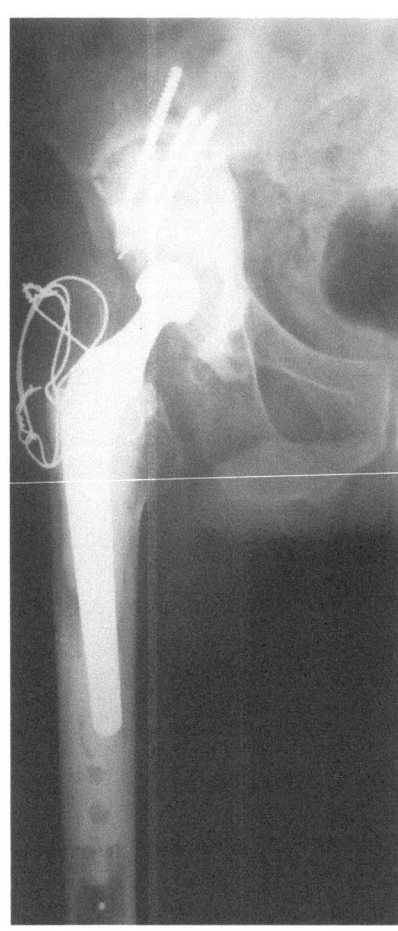

Fig. 9.2 One month after revision with LFA. A frozen
femoral head allograft fixed with three *screws* was used to
fill the spherical defect of the pelvis

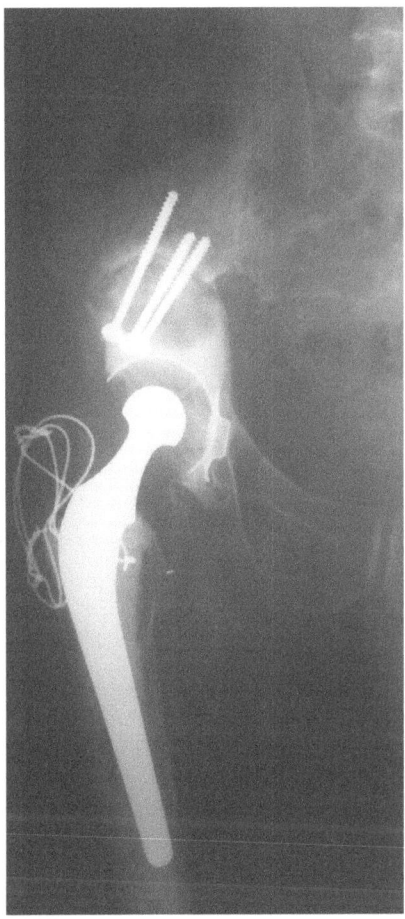

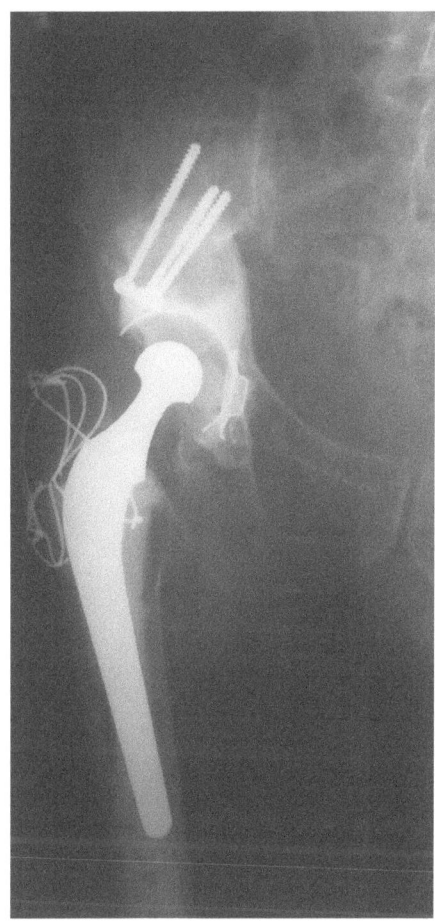

Fig. 9.3 Radiograph, 4 months after revision, the graft had partially resorbed

Fig. 9.4 One year after revision, revascularisation of the graft had started. The patient began to walk with full weight bearing

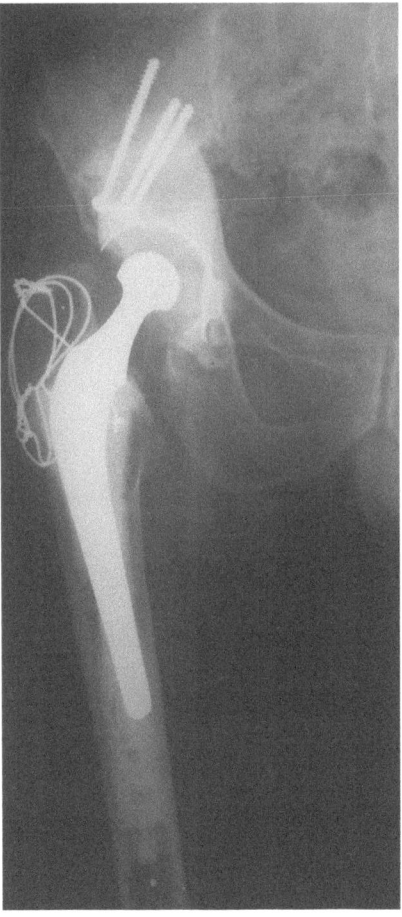

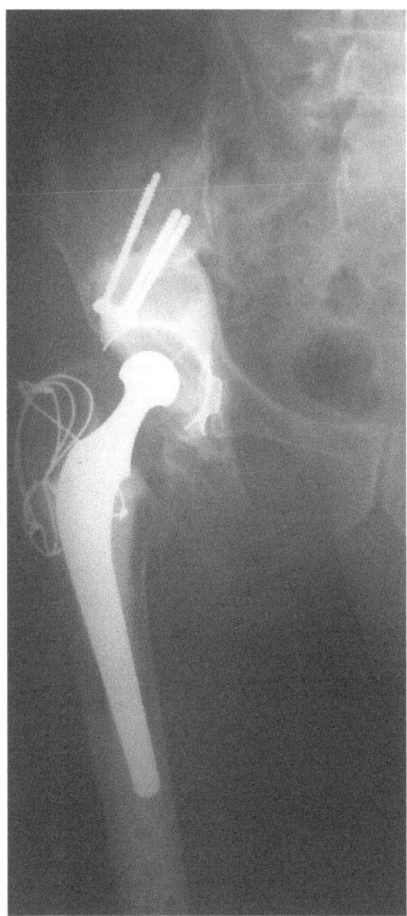

Fig. 9.5 Radiograph 5 years after revision. The graft was fully revascularised and the cup remained stable

Fig. 9.6 The last follow-up radiograph at the tenth post-revision year

9.2 Case 2

This male patient was born in 1947. At the age of 2 years, he started having pain and limping on the right hip. He had no treatment and was slightly limping since then. We first examined him in 1979, when he was 32 years old and hip symptoms had aggravated. Based on patient's history and radiographs, the diagnosis of secondary OA of the right hip due to osteochondritis was made. We performed an LFA.

Since that time, the patient had a painless hip, no limping and a fully active life for many years. At the 21th postoperative year follow-up, in 2000, a significant acetabulum wear was noticed. The patient remained asymptomatic. He was closely followed for the next years with the concern of the development of periprosthetic osteolysis. This was delayed for almost 10 years, when the patient denied our recommendation for acetabular component revision. Revision was finally performed 35 years postoperatively, in 2014, when the patient accepted to be operated, as he had severe hip pain and heavy limping. The acetabulum was completely destroyed and more complicated technique needed for its reconstruction.

At the last follow-up, 2 years after revision, the patient was 69 years old, fully active, and had no hip pain or limping (Figs. 9.7–9.14).

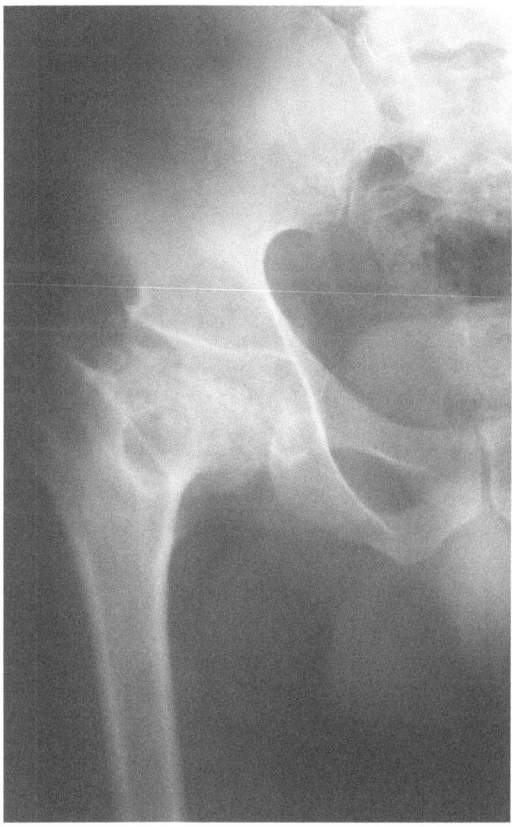

Fig. 9.7 Preoperative radiograph taken in 1979, when the patient was 32 years old. The diagnosis of secondary OA due to osteochondritis was made

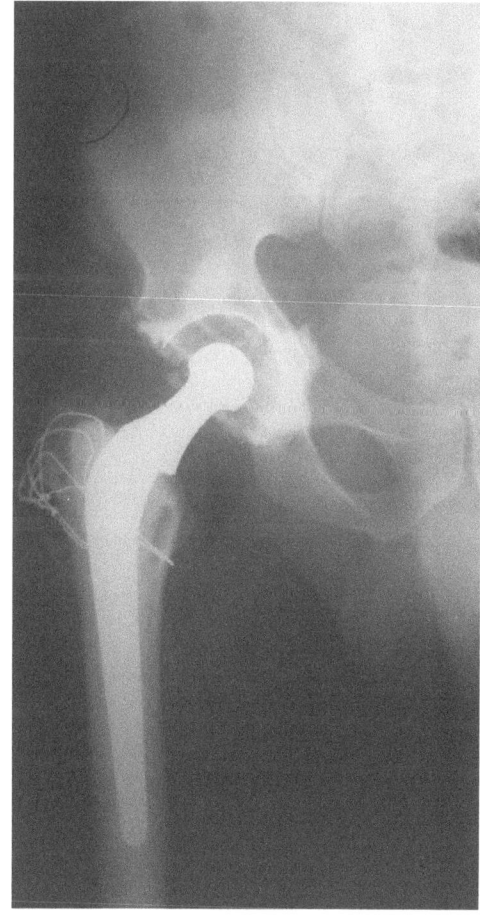

Fig. 9.8 Postoperative radiograph

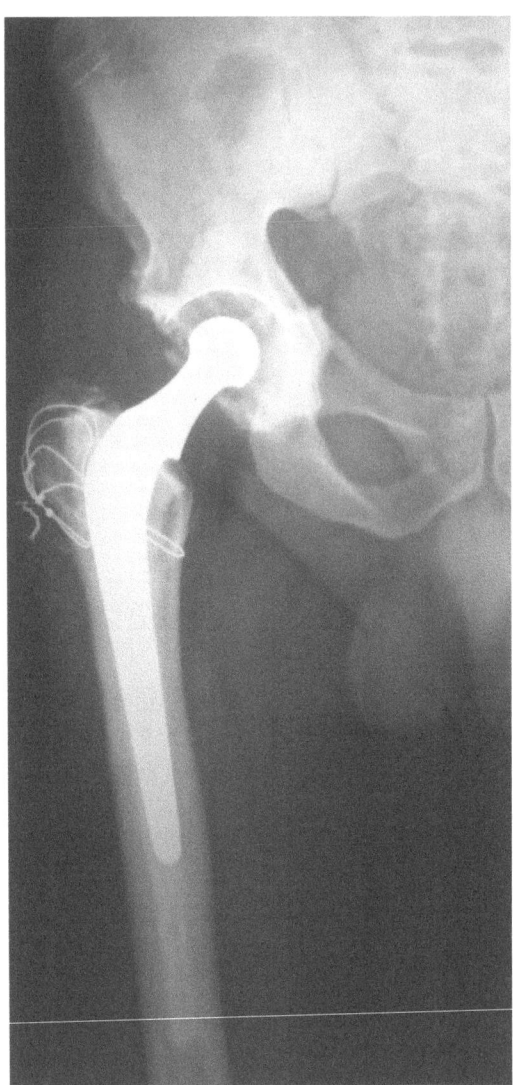

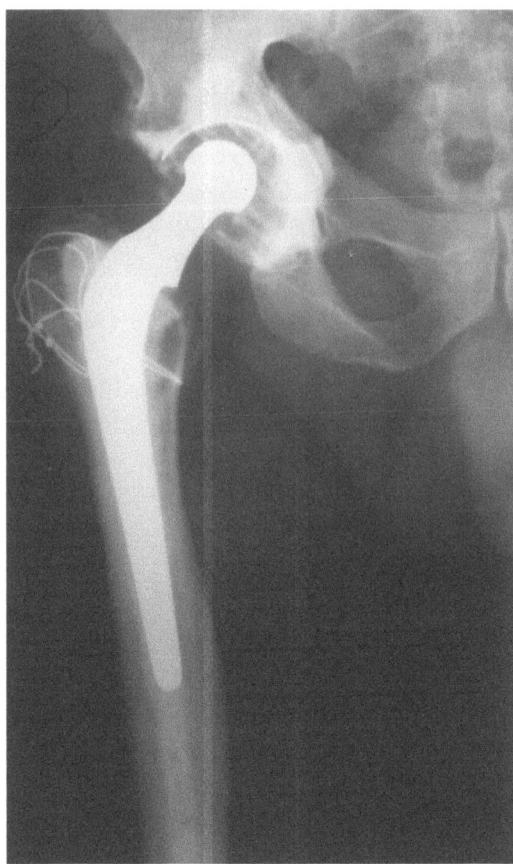

Fig. 9.10 This radiograph was taken 21 years postoperatively in 2000. The acetabulum wear had significantly increased without osteolysis. The patient was asymptomatic

Fig. 9.9 Radiograph 10 years postoperatively, when slight acetabulum wear was first noticed

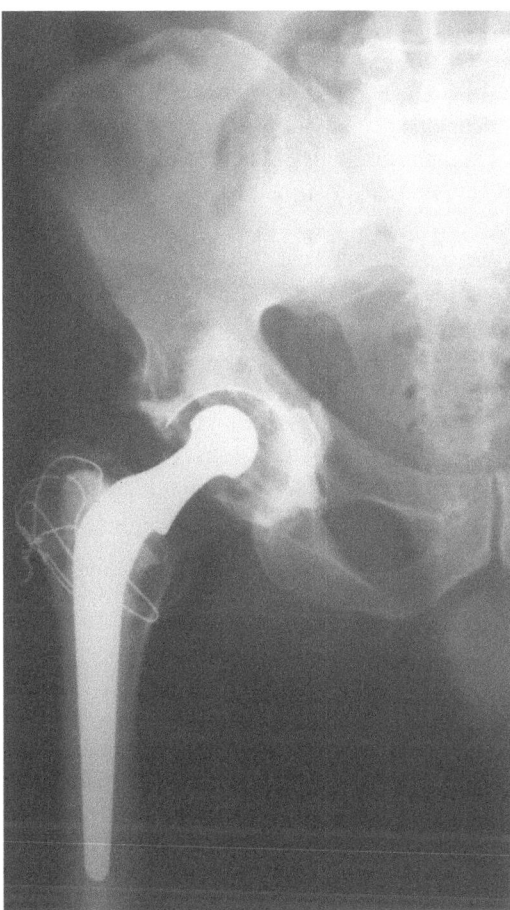 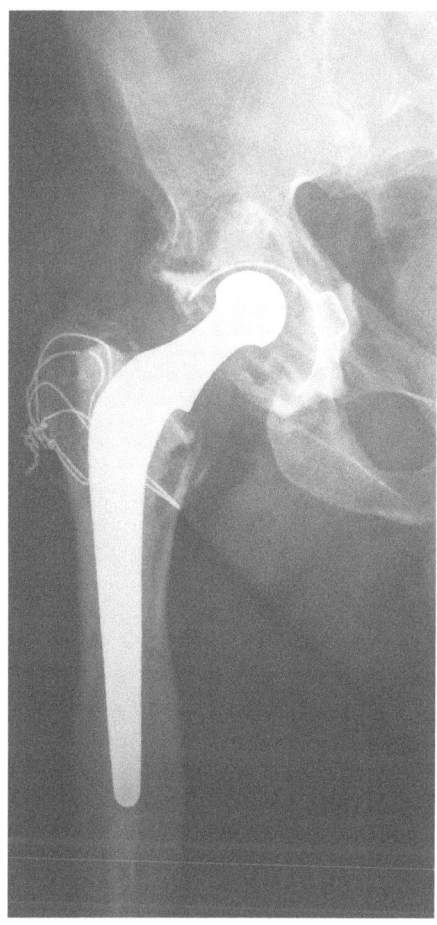

Fig. 9.11 Four years later and 25 years after primary LFA, there is further progression of wear of the acetabulum associated with limited linear osteolysis around the acetabulum

Fig. 9.12 Radiograph taken in 2010, 31 years after replacement, when we recommended acetabular component's revision because of the increased acetabular wear and the expansion of the osteolysis. The patient refused our recommendation

9.3   Case 3

This female patient was born in 1934 with complete dislocation of the right hip. She had no treatment in infancy. At the age of 54 years, she underwent a cemented THR in an institution abroad. The surgeon decided not to osteotomise the greater trochanter. The result was postoperative palsy of the femoral and the peroneal nerve and early loosening of both components.

In 1990, 2 years after primary replacement, we performed a cement-in-cement revision of both components. The result was to get a painless and stable hip, but the nerve function never resolved. The patient was walking for the rest of her life holding a crutch in the contralateral hand. She died in 2012, 78 years old, from reason unrelated to THR (Figs. 9.15–9.18).

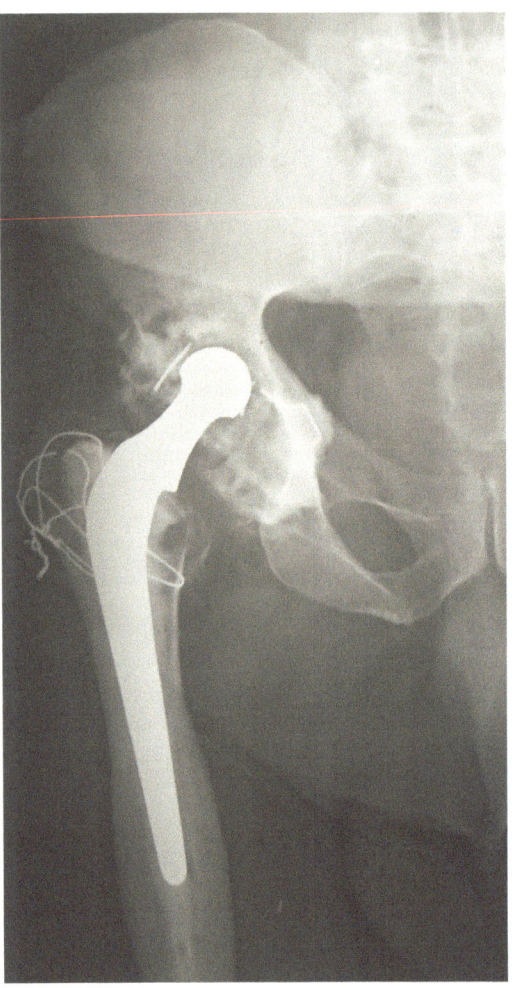

Fig. 9.13 This radiograph was taken 4 years later, 35 years postoperatively, when the patient agreed to undergo revision

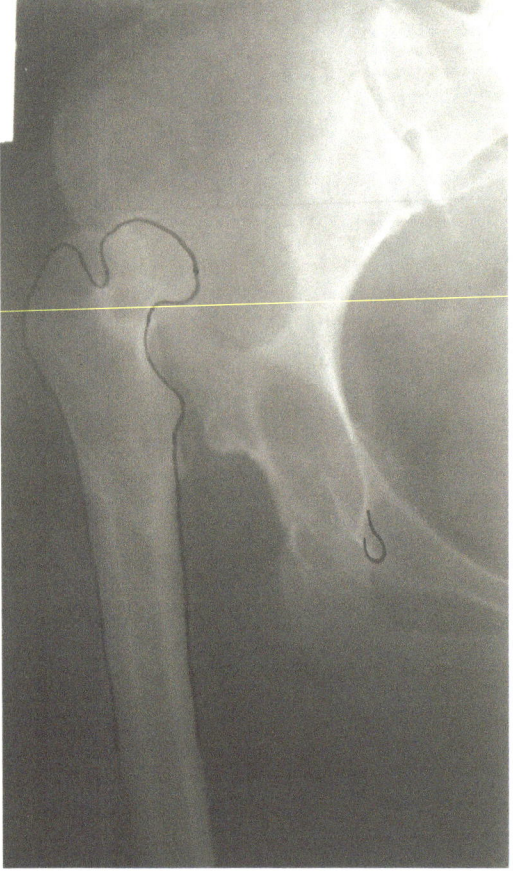

Fig. 9.15 Radiograph before the primary replacement

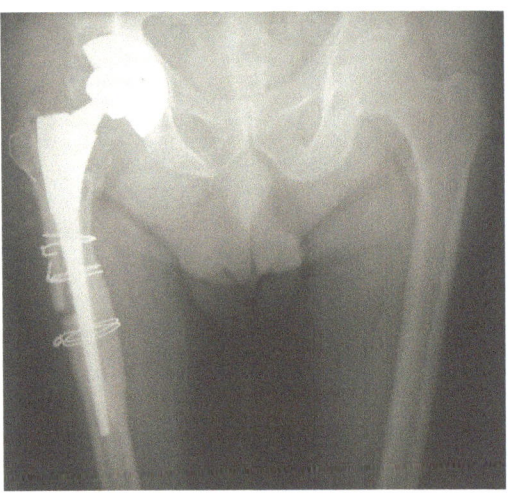

Fig. 9.14 The last follow-up radiograph taken 1 year after revision of both components

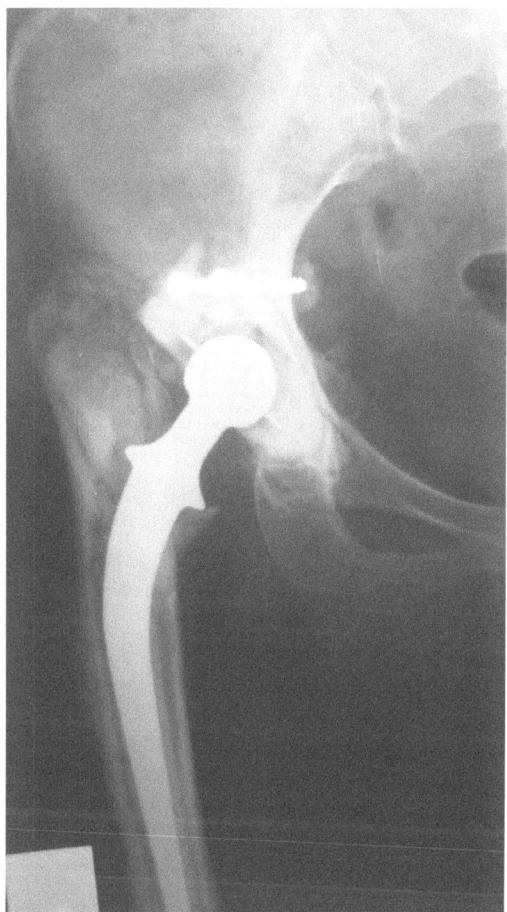

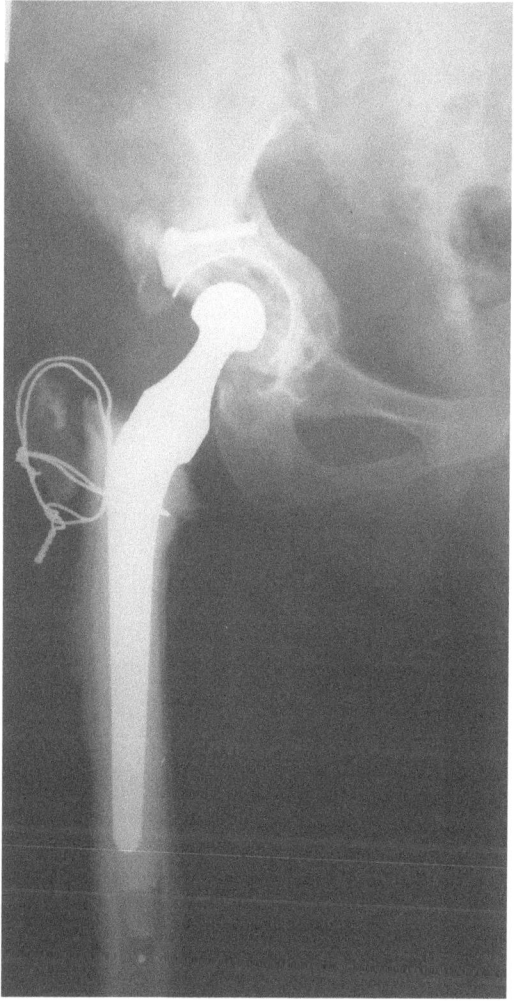

Fig. 9.16 Two years postoperatively. There was loosening of both components. The patient had hip pain and severe limping mostly because of femoral and peroneal nerve palsies

Fig. 9.17 Early post-revision radiograph

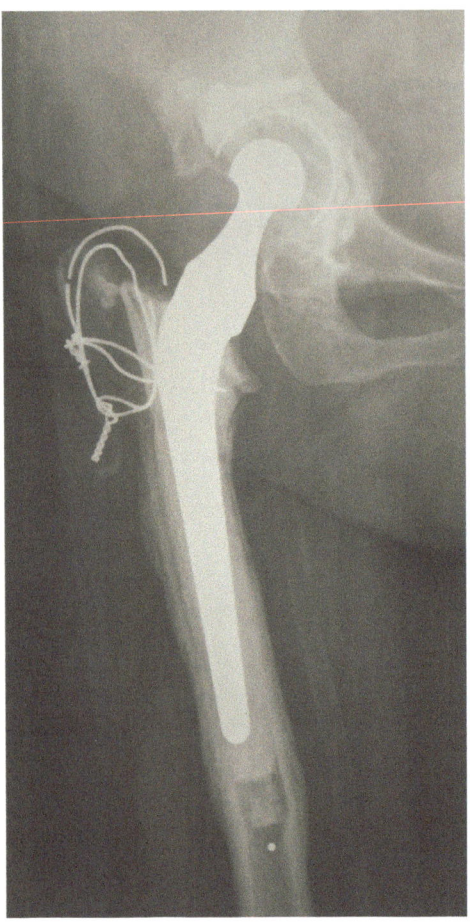

Fig. 9.18 The latest follow-up radiograph that was taken 12 years after revision. She died 10 years later

9.4 Case 4

This female patient was born in 1934 with bilateral CHD. She had no treatment in infancy. She was limping since then. We first examined her, in 1977, at the age of 43 years. She had severe disability because of secondary OA due to low dislocation of both hips. We performed LFA of the right hip, as it was more painful. Soon after the replacement, Brooker grade 4 heterotopic ossification was developed, resulting in complete ankylosis of the hip in 20° of flexion and 20° of external rotation. Operation of the left hip was postponed with the concern that heterotopic ossification may also develop.

Removal of heterotopic ossification was attempted 20 years later, in 1997, resulting in the mobilisation of the joint, which gained 70° of flexion, 15° of abduction and 10° of adduction. External rotation ranged from 15° to 20°. Since this result was maintained, 1 year later, THR of the left hip was decided. At the last follow-up, 39 and 18 years after THR of the right and left hip, respectively, the patient, at the age of 82 years, had limited indoor activities mainly because of symptoms of severe spinal stenosis (Figs. 9.19–9.24).

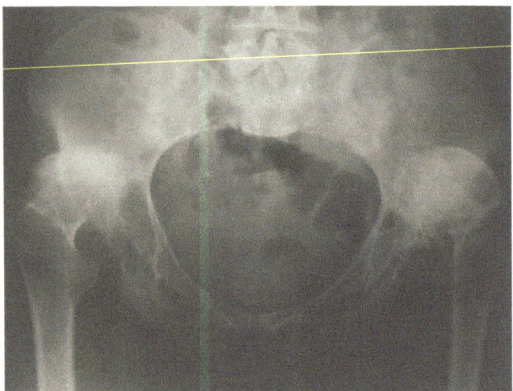

Fig. 9.19 Preoperative radiograph, when the patient was 43 years old

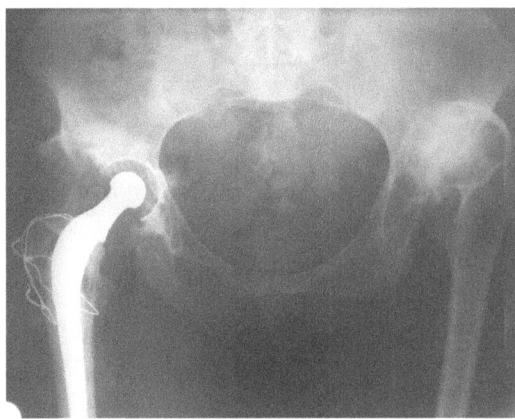

Fig. 9.20 Forty-five days after LFA of the right hip. The first signs of the development of heterotopic ossification appeared

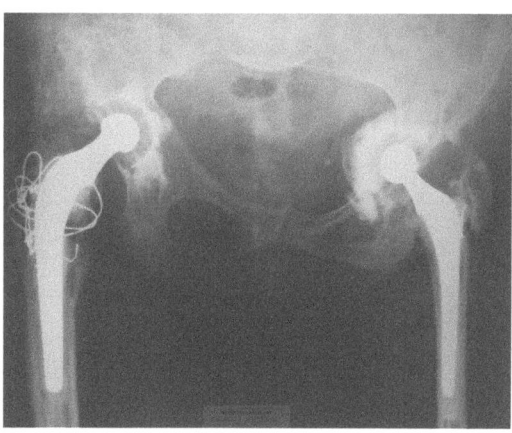

Fig. 9.23 This radiograph was taken 3 years after removal of the greater part of heterotopic bone of the right hip and 2 years after left THR

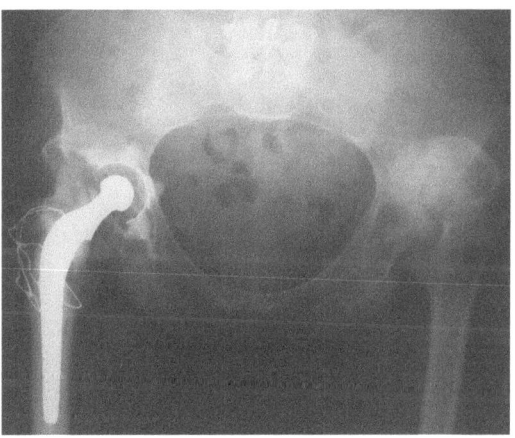

Fig. 9.21 Eighteen months postoperatively, Brooker grade 4 heterotopic ossification had been developed

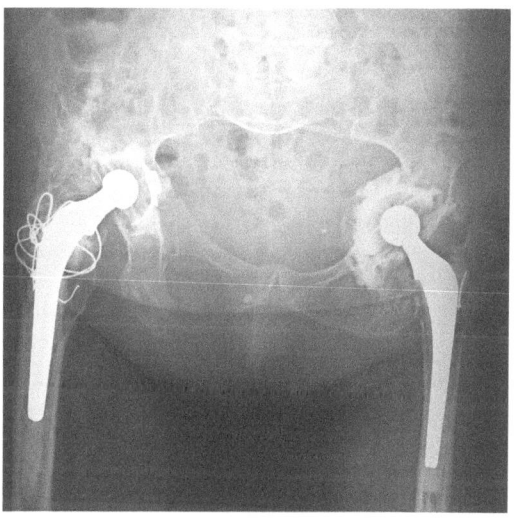

Fig. 9.24 The latest available radiograph, 39 and 18 years after right and left THR, respectively

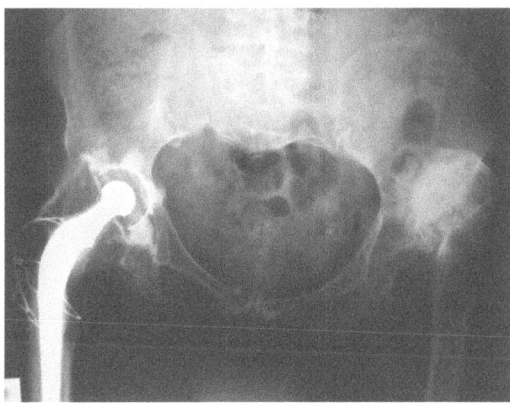

Fig. 9.22 Radiograph taken in 1997, 20 years after primary replacement, before removal of heterotopic bone

9.5   Case 5

This male patient was born in 1931. At the age of 54 years, he had a severe traffic accident and had been treated for 3 years in different hospitals. When he was admitted to our department, in 1988, he had three main problems: (1) nonunion of the right femoral neck fracture with AVN of the femoral head, (2) malunion of the left femoral fracture and (3) septic nonunion of the left tibia.

We decided to treat first the left tibia with external fixation and repeated surgical debridements, and then the right hip with LFA, despite the increased risk of periprosthetic joint infection. We accepted the malunion of the left femoral shaft fracture. THR remained free of complications, but the left tibia, although the fracture had been fused, maintained with chronic osteomyelitis. The following years, there was functional improvement, and at the last follow-up examination, 28 years after primary right THR, the patient at the age of 85 years had satisfactory activities compatible to his age without having hip pain (Figs. 9.25–9.29).

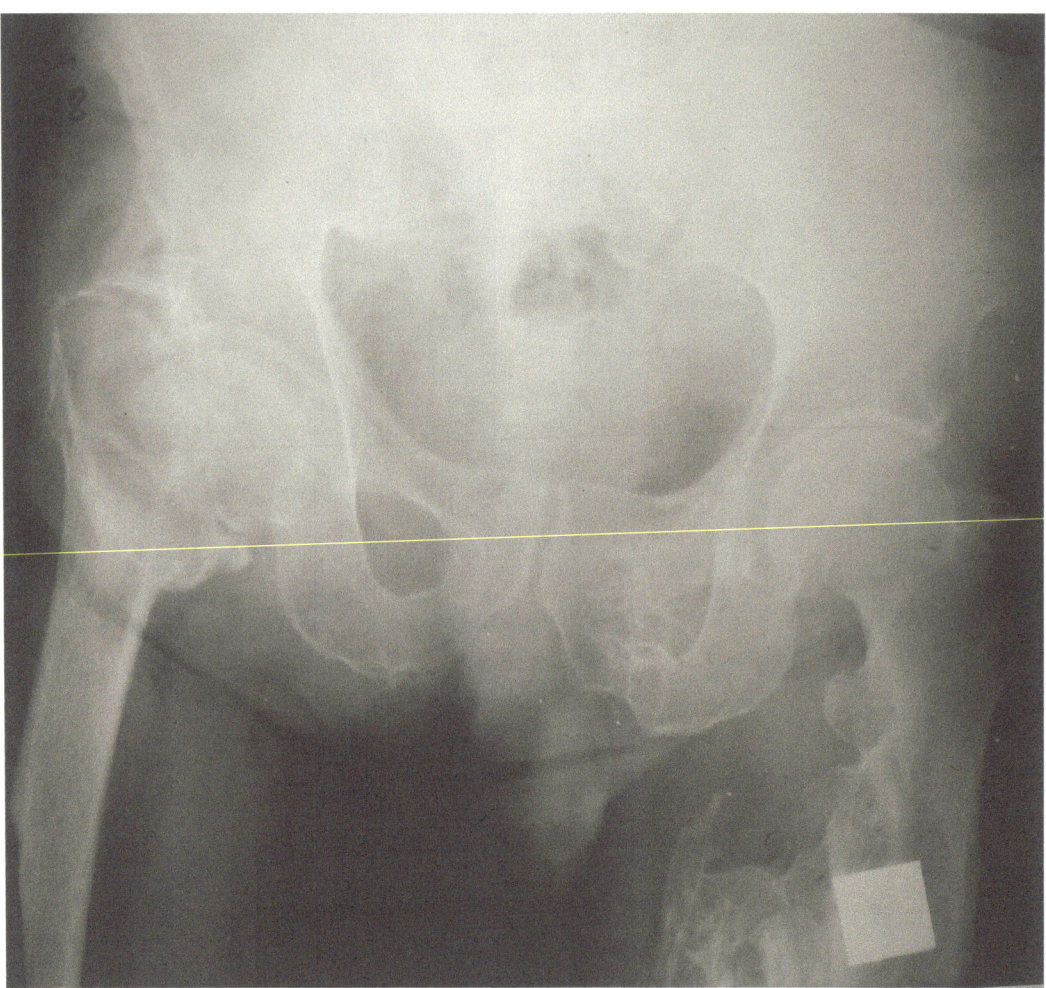

Fig. 9.25 Radiograph of the pelvis, at patient's admission to the hospital in 1988. Note the nonunion of the right femoral neck fracture and the malunion of the left femoral fracture

Fig. 9.26 (**a**) Anteroposterior and (**b**) lateral radiographs of the left tibia, at patient's admission to the hospital. The diagnosis of septic nonunion was made

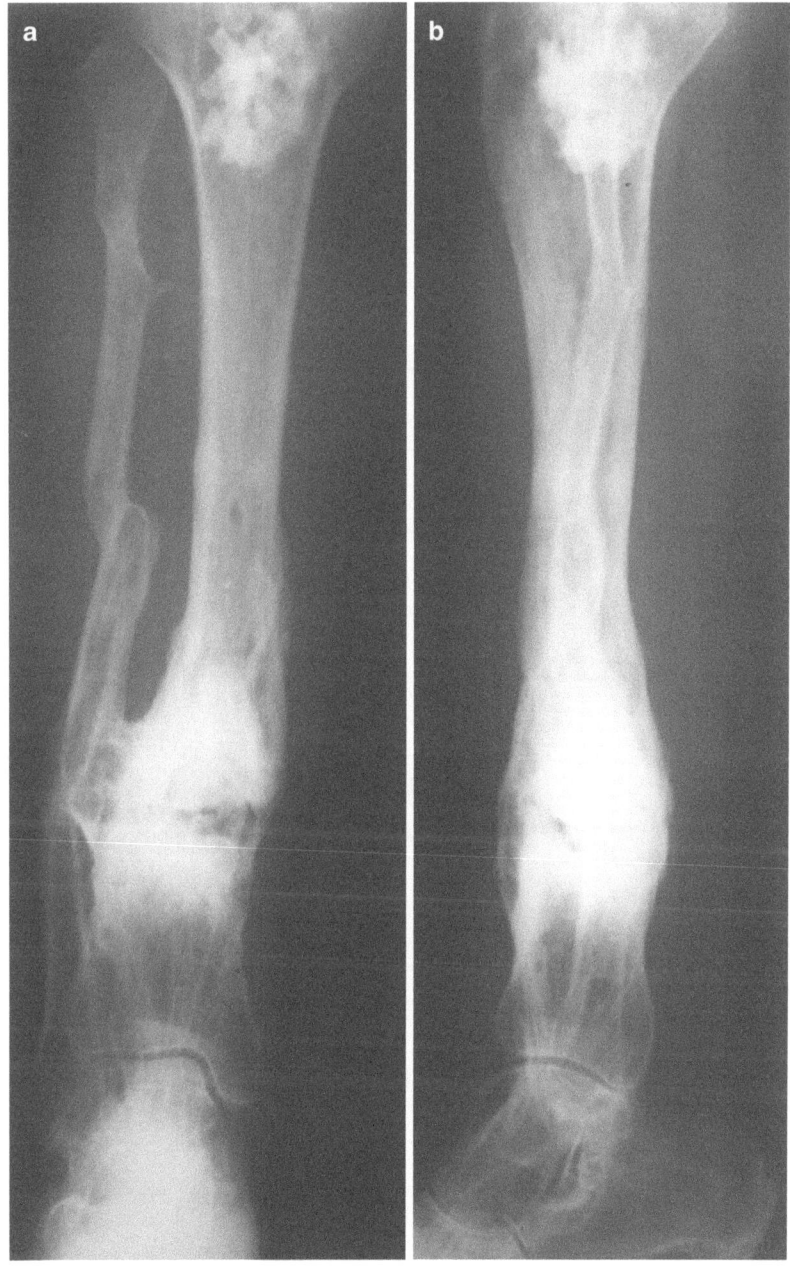

Fig. 9.27 Three months after right LFA

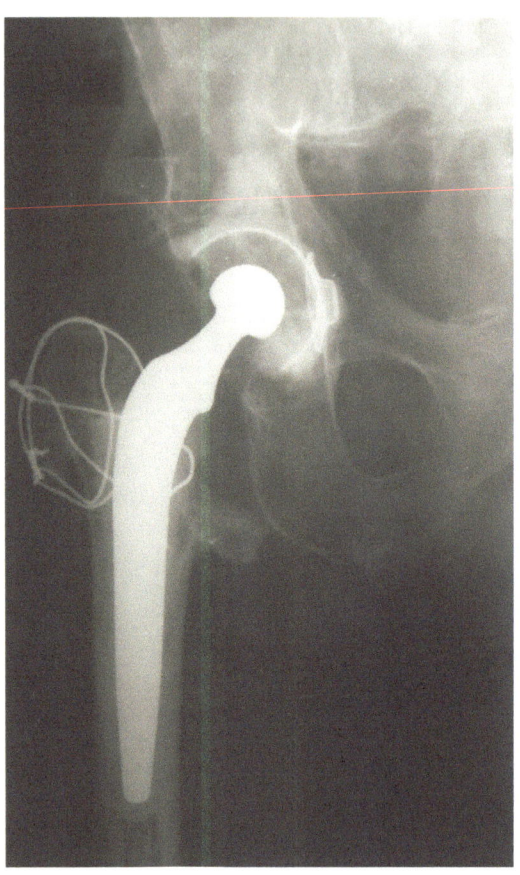

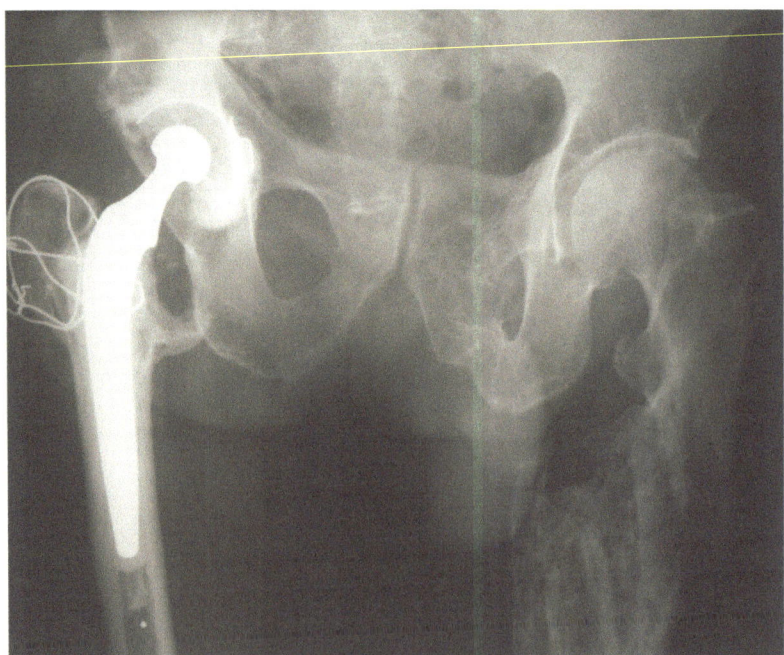

Fig. 9.28 The latest
follow-up radiograph was
taken 28 years after
primary THR

Fig. 9.29 (a) Anteroposterior and (b) lateral radiographs of the left tibia at the patient's latest examination. Despite the union of the fracture of the tibia, chronic osteomyelitis remained

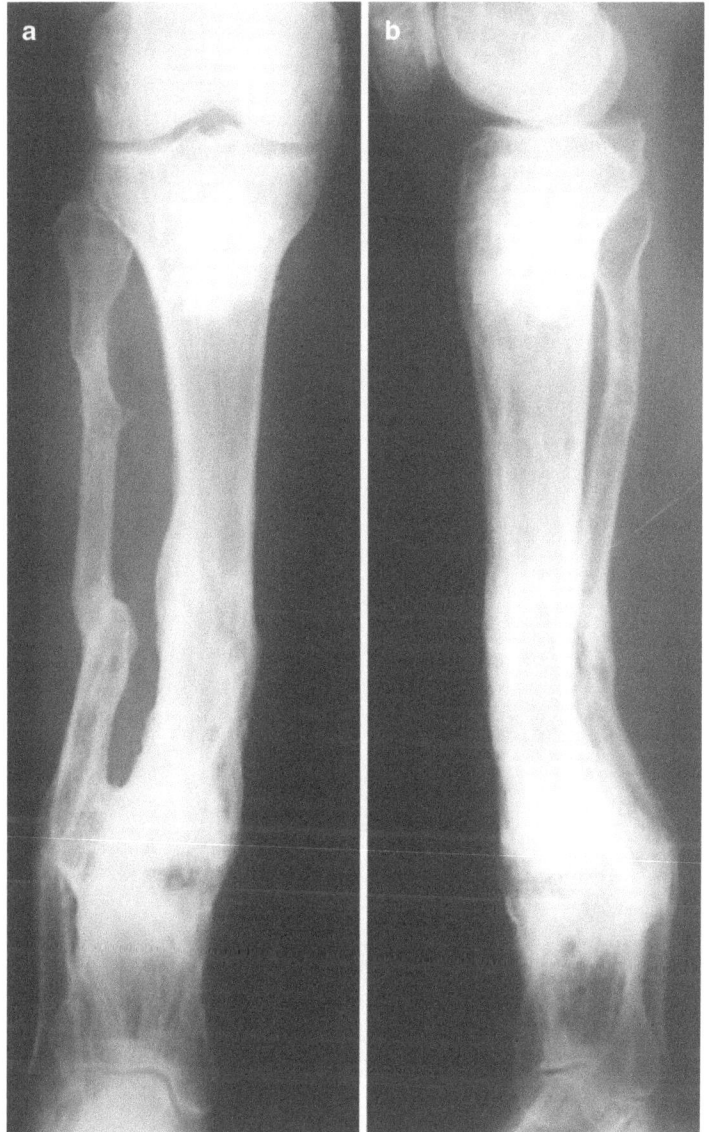

9.6   Case 6

This female patient was born in 1939 with congenital disease of the right hip. She had no treatment in infancy. She was limping, but the pain started around the age of 20 years. The development of secondary OA of the hip, classified as having low dislocation, was slow. THR was performed when the patient was 51 years old, in 1990.

At the age of 65 years, in 2004, she started having pain in the left hip because of the development of idiopathic OA. Deterioration of this hip was rapid and THR was needed within 3 years. The latest radiographic follow-up was performed 26 and 9 years after primary right and left THR, respectively. The patient was 77 years old, fully active and free of hip pain (Figs. 9.30–9.35).

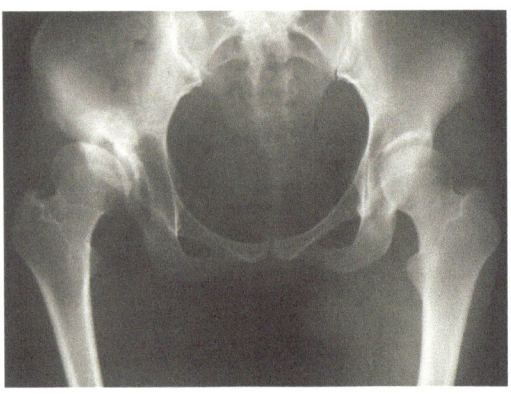

Fig. 9.30 Radiograph taken in 1963 when the patient was 24 years old. The right hip had low dislocation with onset of secondary OA and the left hip was normal

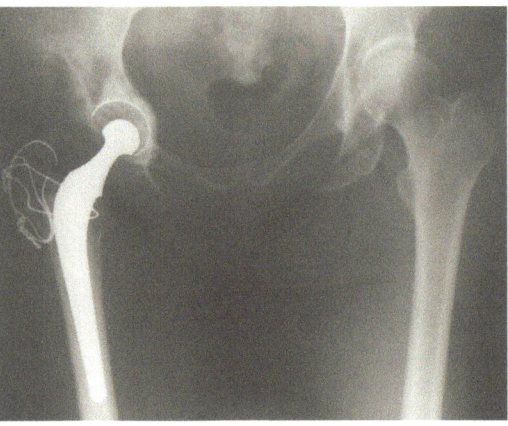

Fig. 9.32 Radiograph 2 years after LFA. Note that the left hip was normal

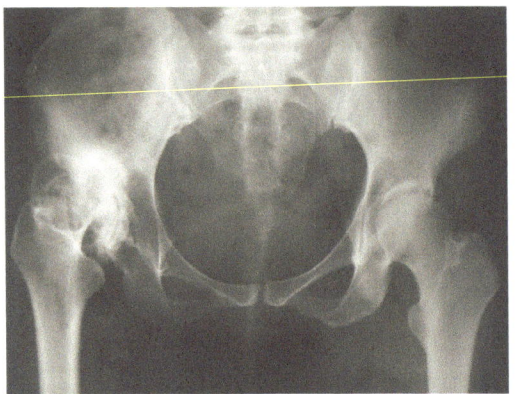

Fig. 9.31 Radiograph 25 years later, in 1988, when the patient consulted us because pain and limping on the right hip had aggravated. THR was followed

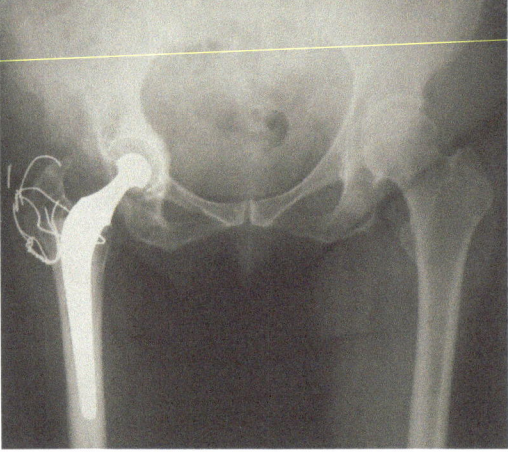

Fig. 9.33 At the age of 65 years, 14 years after replacement of the right hip, the patient started having pain in the left hip because of the onset of eccentric idiopathic OA

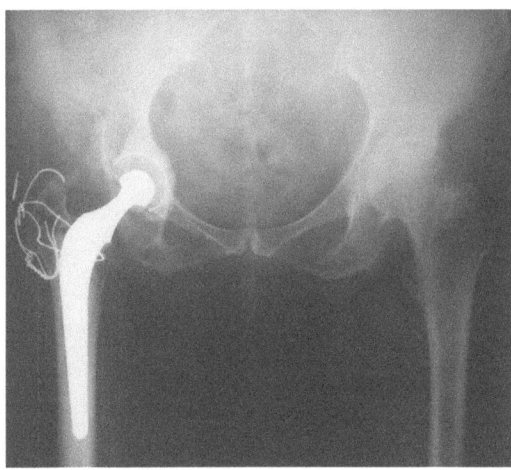

Fig. 9.34 Rapid deterioration of the left hip made the THR necessary after 3 years, in 2007

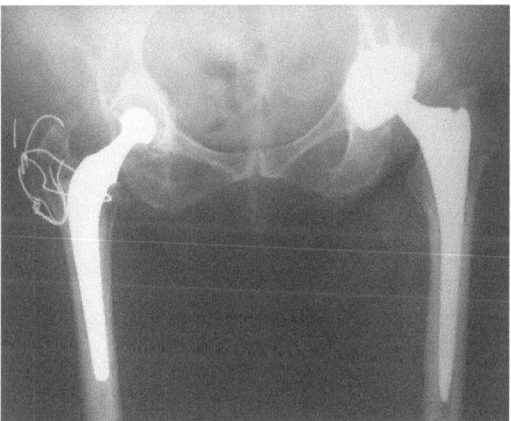

Fig. 9.35 The last follow-up radiograph 26 and 9 years after right and left primary THR, respectively

9.7   Cases 7, 8 and 9

Three generations of females of the same family with CHD.

9.7.1   Case 7

She is the mother of the patient described in Case 8 and the grandmother of the patient described in Case 9. She was born in 1912 with CHD of both hips. We performed, in 1963, a proximal femoral osteotomy supported by Nissen combined with the Voss operation of the left hip and, in 1967, a varus osteotomy of the right. LFA of the left hip was needed, in 1974, when the patient was 62 years old and of the right, in 1989, when the patient was 77 years old. Twenty-six years after LFA of the left hip, in 2000, the stem fractured, but the patient remained without any further treatment, because of bad general health. She died 2 years later at the age of 90 years (Figs. 9.36–9.39).

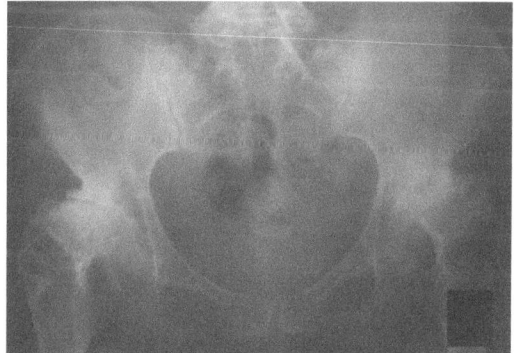

Fig. 9.36 Radiograph before left THR, taken in 1974, when the patient was 62 years old. The left hip was classified as having dysplasia and the right as having low dislocation. Previous osteotomies of the left and right hip had been performed 11 and 7 years, respectively

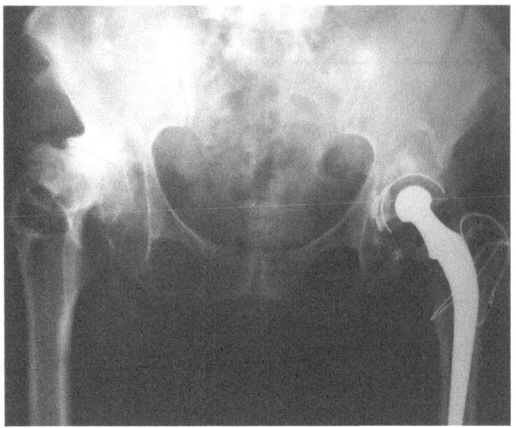

Fig. 9.37 Eight years after LFA of the left hip

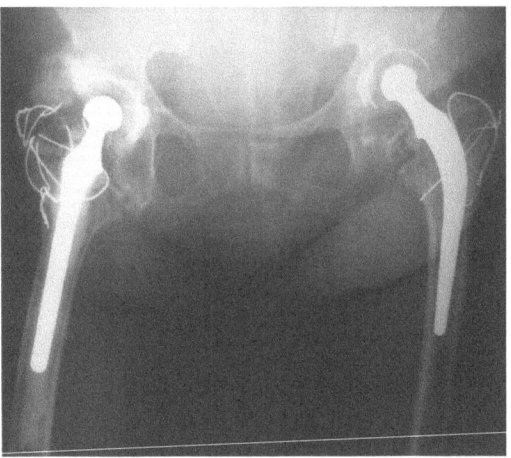

Fig. 9.38 This radiograph was taken in 1999, 25 and 10 years after LFA of the left and right hip, respectively

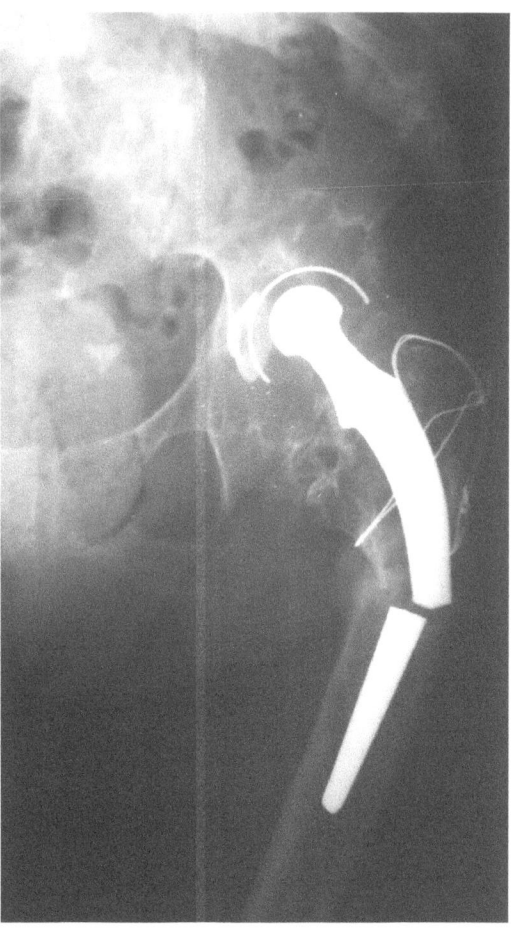

Fig. 9.39 One year later, stem of the left hip was fractured. The patient remained without further treatment, because of bad general condition and died 2 years later at the age of 90 years

9.7.2 Case 8

She is the daughter of the patient described in Case 7 and the mother of the patient described in Case 9. She was born in 1948. She started having slight limping and occasional mild pain in the right hip since adolescence. She was 17 years old, in 1965, when we diagnosed that the right hip was dysplastic without OA changes.

A varus osteotomy was performed. She remained without hip pain for many years. She got married and had two daughters. Pain and limping started around the age of 45 years, and we performed a hybrid THR, 31 years after the varus osteotomy, in 1996, when she was 48 years old. For the next 20 years, until the last follow-up examination, she was free of symptoms and had a normal life (Figs. 9.40–9.46).

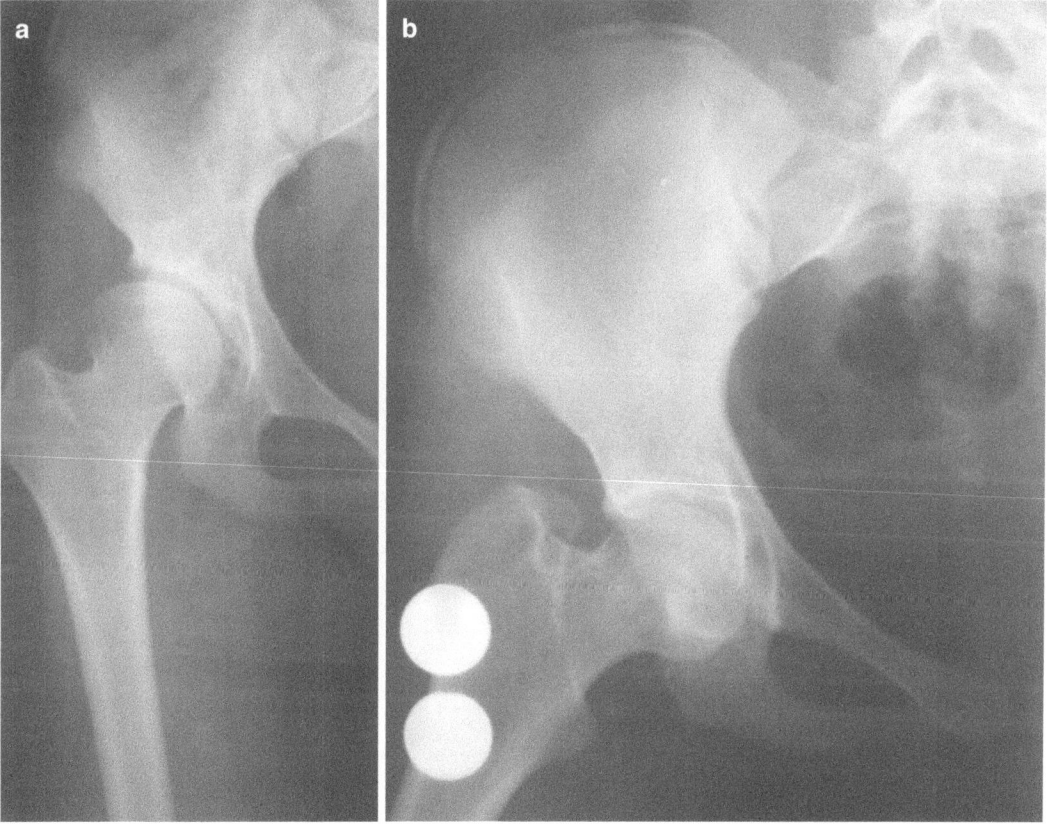

Fig. 9.40 (**a**) Radiograph of the dysplastic right hip, when the patient was 17 years old. (**b**) Radiograph in abduction showed complete coverage of the femoral head and congruity of the articular surfaces

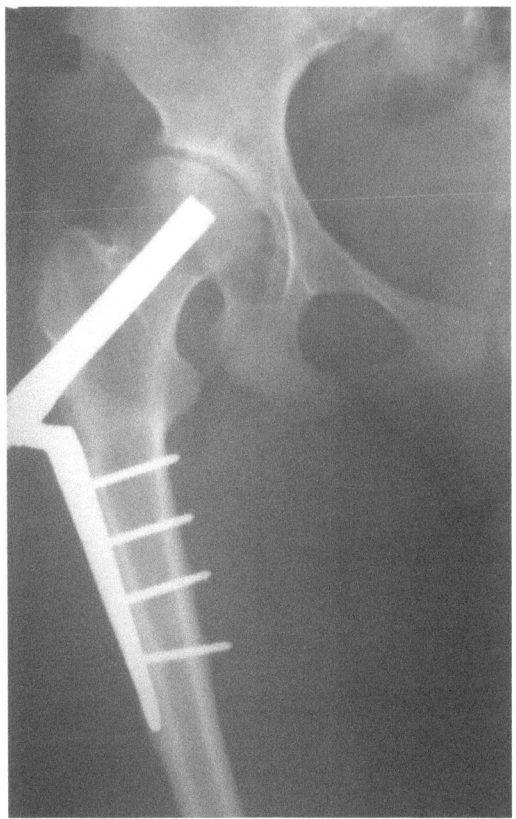

Fig. 9.41 Radiograph after varus osteotomy

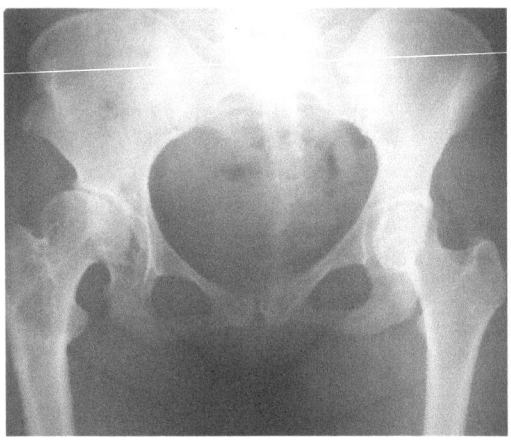

Fig. 9.42 Ten years post-osteotomy

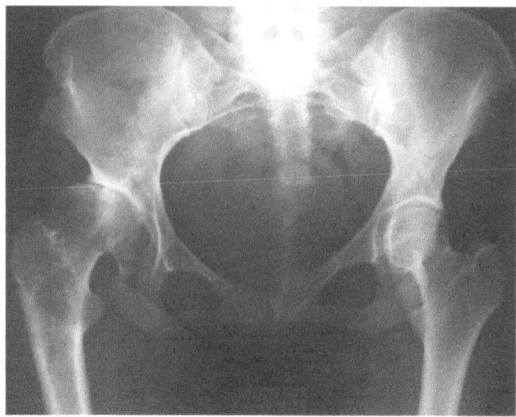

Fig. 9.43 Twenty years post-osteotomy. The patient remained asymptomatic

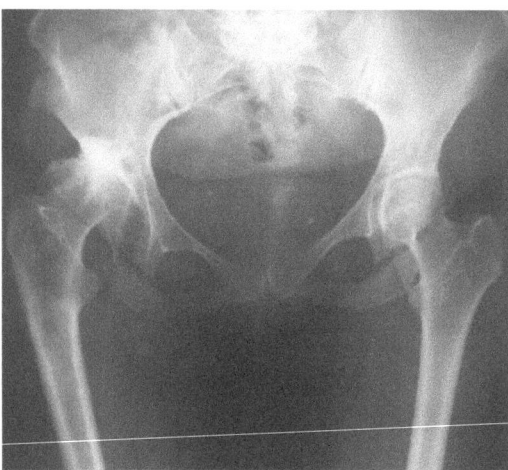

Fig. 9.44 Radiograph 31 years after osteotomy, in 1996, when THR was decided

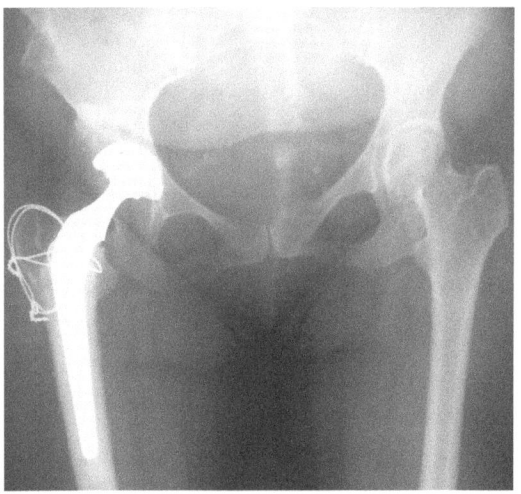

Fig. 9.45 Radiograph after hybrid THR, when the patient was 48 years old

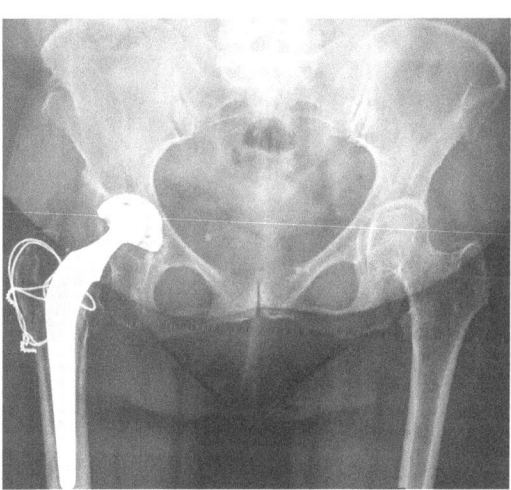

Fig. 9.46 The final follow-up radiograph was taken 20 years after THR, when the patient was 68 years old

9.7.3   Case 9

She is the daughter of the patient described in Case 8 and the granddaughter of the patient described in Case 7. She was born in 1984. She underwent early radiographic evaluation, at the age of 3 months, because of the familial history. Suspicious signs of CHD of both hips led us to treat her with application of an abduction pillow. The patient was followed until the age of 8 years, and, possibly owing to the early diagnosis and the proper treatment, she had normal development of both hips (Figs. 9.47–9.49).

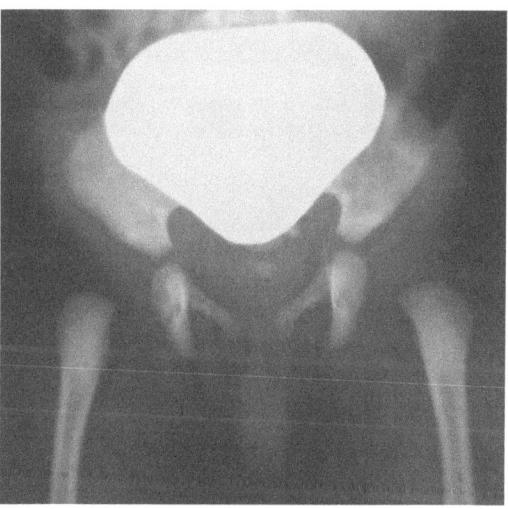

Fig. 9.47 Radiograph when the infant was 3 months old. The ossific nuclei of the femoral heads are not yet evident. There is increased acetabular index and lateral displacement of the femurs in both hips, more pronounced in the right. The Shenton's line seems to be disrupted. An abduction pillow was applied

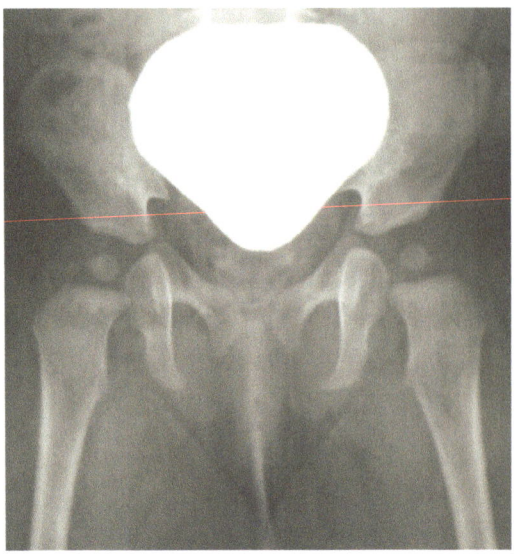

Fig. 9.48 This radiograph was taken when the patient was 13 months old. The normal development of both hips was maintained

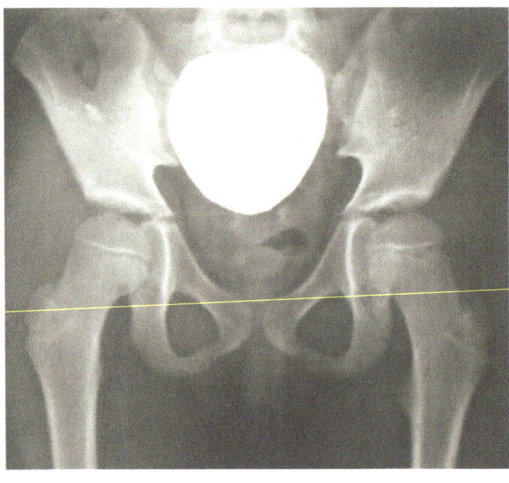

Fig. 9.49 At the latest follow-up, at the age of 8 years. The normal development of both hips was confirmed

9.8   Case 10

This female patient was born in 1961 with congenital disease of the left hip. At the age of 2 years, her physician treated her with closed reduction and immobilisation in plaster. She was limping since then, and around the age of 25 years, she started to have hip pain. At the age of 29 years, she underwent cemented THR in another institution and had inadequate follow-up. She was referred to us, 4 years later, with pain and severe limping, in 1994. The reconstruction was difficult, especially because of the complete absence of the outer cortex of the proximal femur. A long stem was used with distal cemented fixation. Twenty-one years after revision, prostheses remained stable, and the patient, at the age of 54 years, remained asymptomatic and had a normal and active life (Figs. 9.50–9.53).

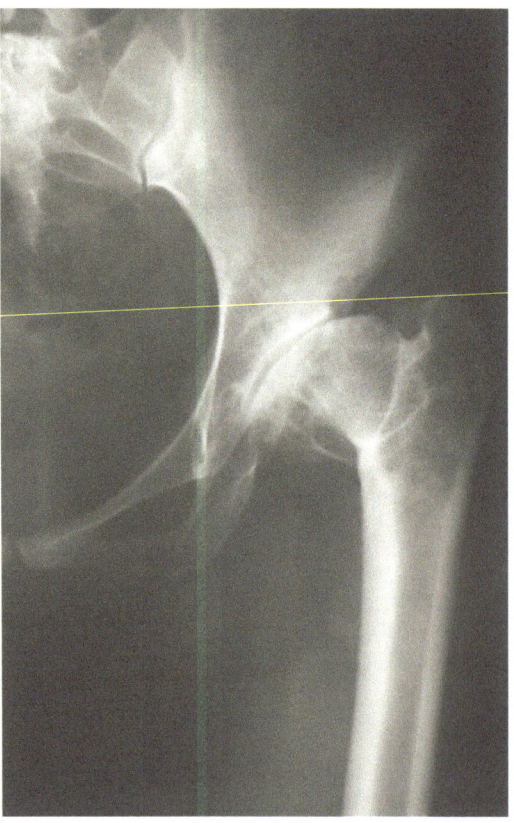

Fig. 9.50 Radiograph that was taken before the primary replacement. The patient had only light discomfort and THR could be postponed with the patient in close observation. However, THR was decided by her physician

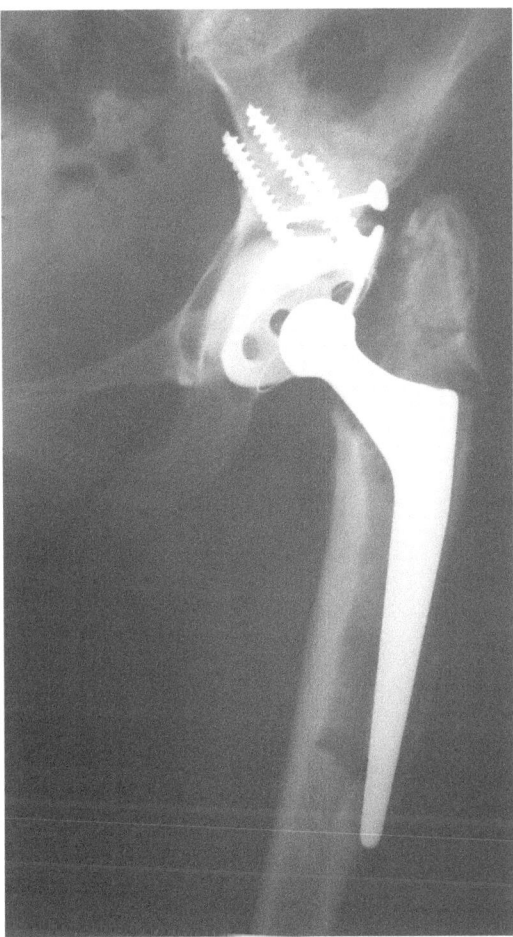

Fig. 9.51 The result of inadequate follow-up. This radiograph was taken when the patient referred to us 4 years after primary replacement

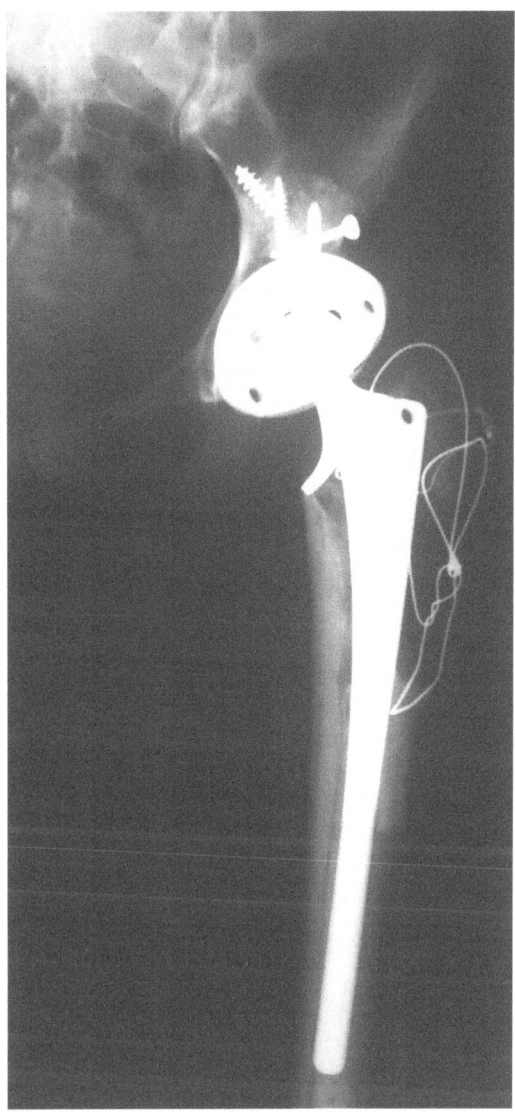

Fig. 9.52 Post-revision radiograph. Note the distal cemented fixation of the long stem

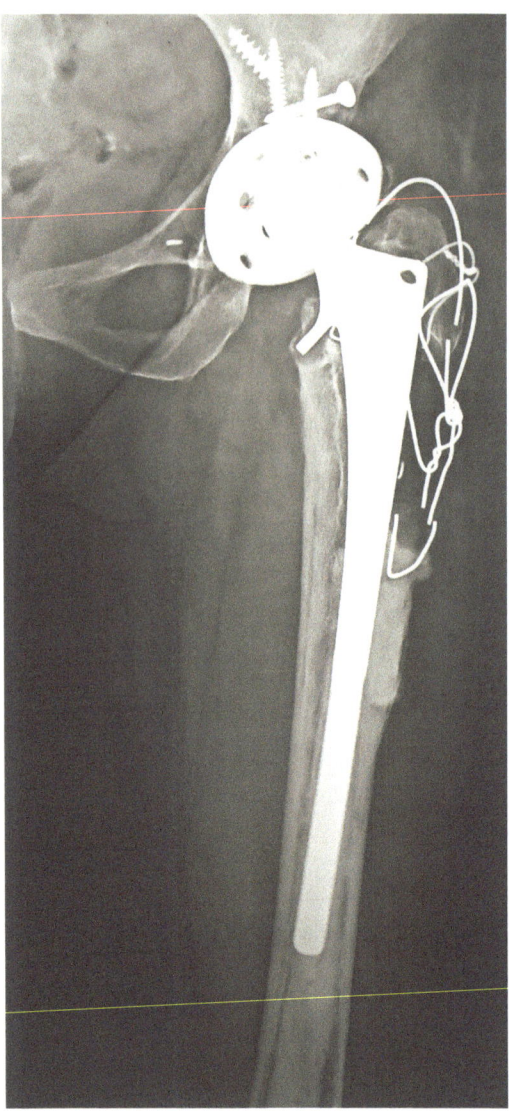

Fig. 9.53 The most recent radiograph was taken 21 years after revision. Satisfactory fixation of implants remained associated with pain-free normal life

9.9   Case 11

This female patient was born in 1921. At the age of 60 years, she had a fracture of the left femoral neck and was treated by her physician with a Bousquet endoprosthesis. There was inadequate follow-up. She referred to us, 5 years later, in 1986. She had an extended osteolysis of the proximal femur associated with patient's heavy limping and severe hip pain. We performed revision with a long cemented Charnley stem. Presently, 30 years after revision, the patient is 95 years old, and remains free of hip symptoms with activity compatible to her age (Figs. 9.54–9.57).

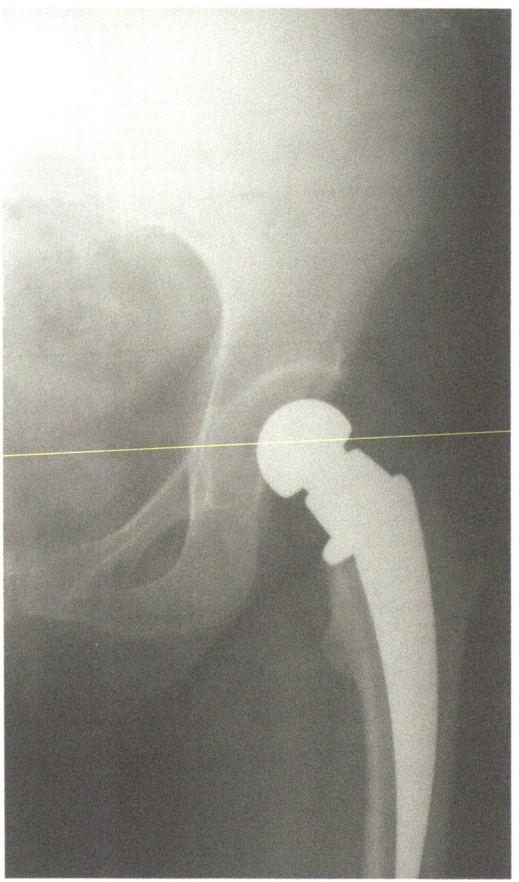

Fig. 9.54 Early radiograph after implantation of Bousquet endoprosthesis

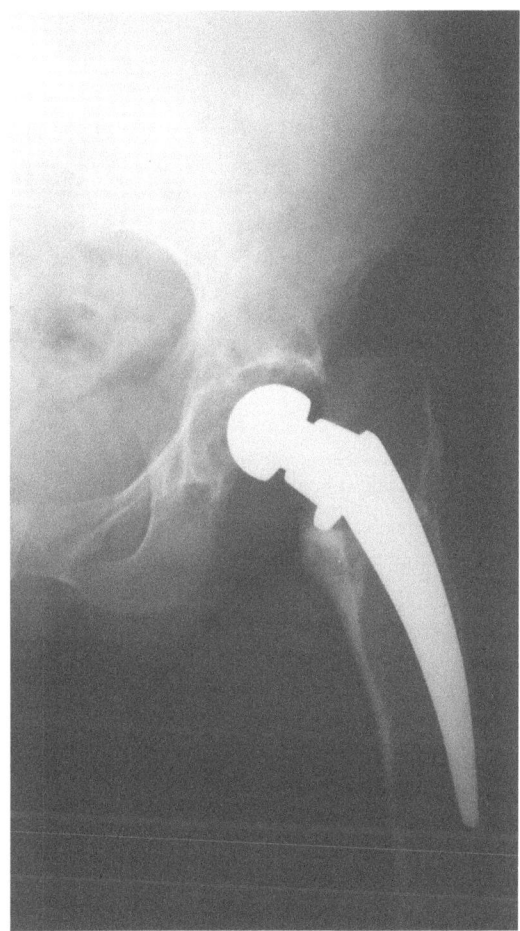

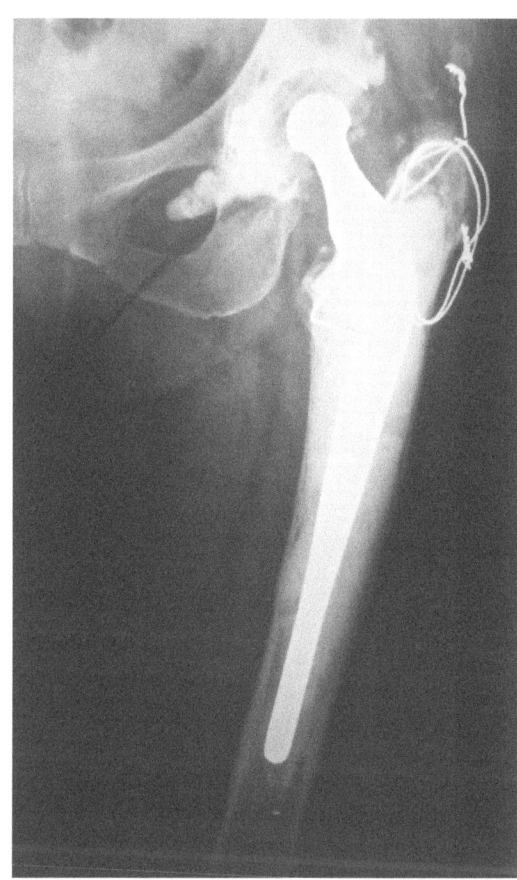

Fig. 9.56 Radiograph, 5 years after cemented revision replacement

Fig. 9.55 Five years later (no intermitted radiographs were taken). Note the extended femoral osteolysis

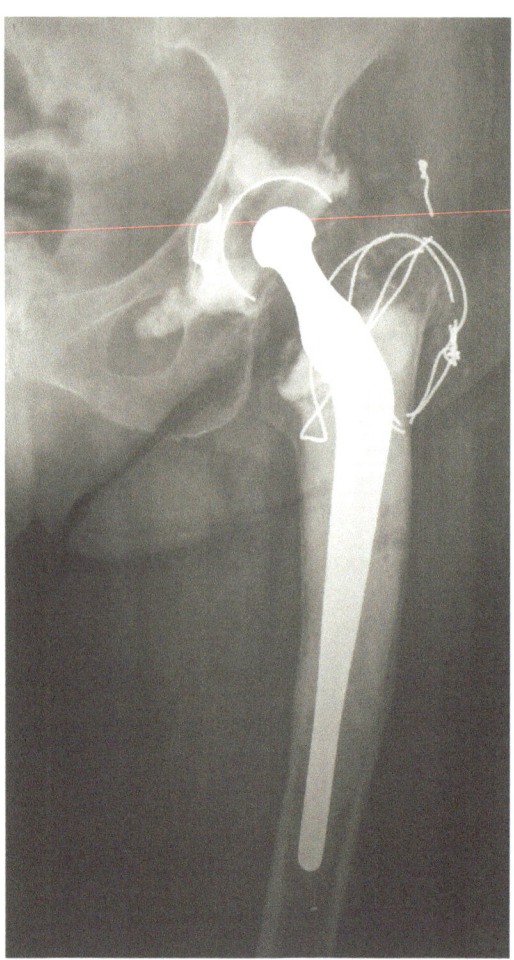

Fig. 9.57 The latest available follow-up radiograph, 24 years post-revision

9.10   Case 12

This female patient was born in 1960. At the age of 4 years, she was treated for congenital subluxation of both hips with a Chiary pelvic osteotomy, according to patient's report, by Chiary himself. She was limping since then, but pain started around the age of 25 years. Gradual aggravation of symptoms followed. Cementless THR of both hips within 10 months was performed by us when the patient was 36 years old. Eleven years after primary THR, isolated polyethylene liner exchange of the right hip was needed. Twenty years later, at the latest follow-up, she was 56 years old, and she had no hip pain. She had normal activities with only slight limping on the right side (Figs. 9.58–9.63).

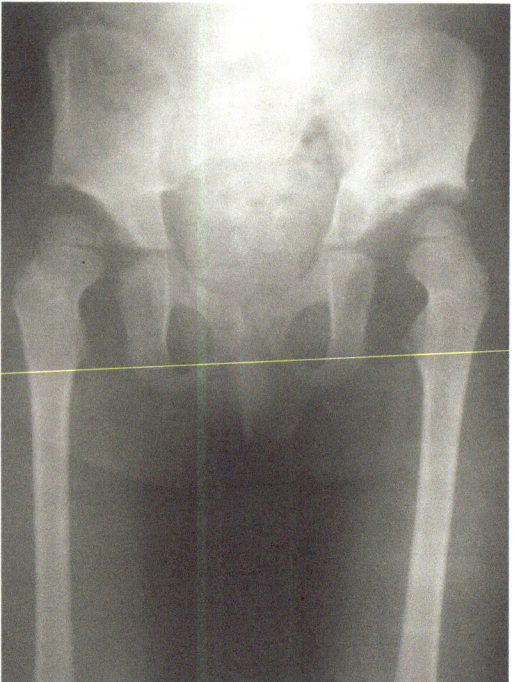

Fig. 9.58 One year after Chiary osteotomies, when the patient was 5 years old

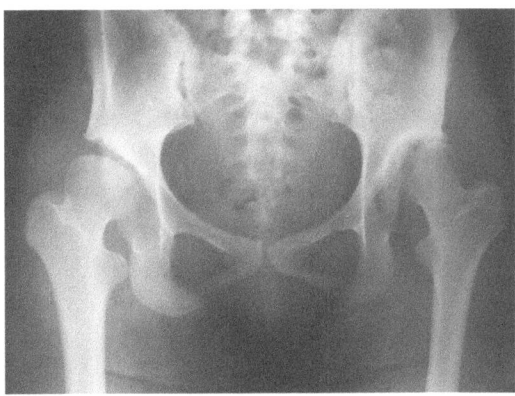

Fig. 9.59   Radiograph at the age of 13 years

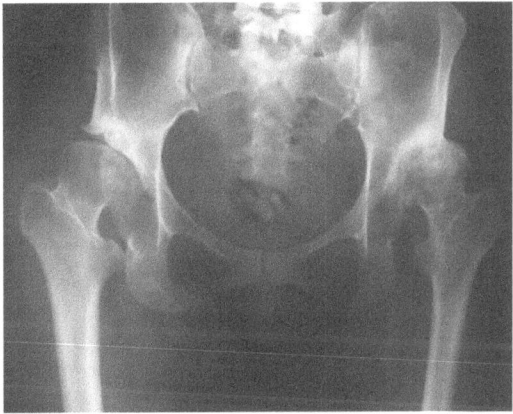

Fig. 9.60   Radiograph, when the patient was 36 years old, before implantation of THRs. The hips had developed low dislocation

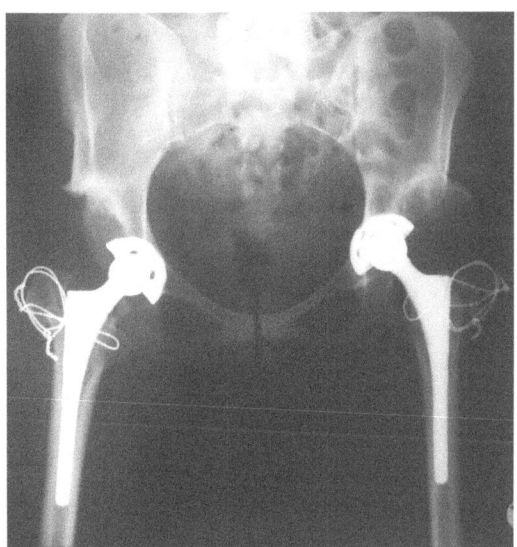

Fig. 9.61   Early radiograph after THRs

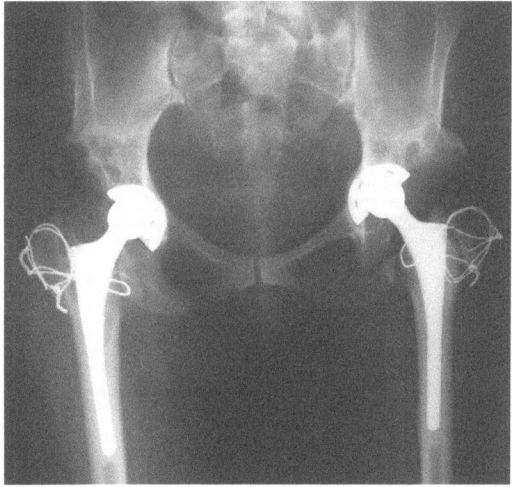

Fig. 9.62   Eleven years after primary THRs. Progressive polyethylene liner wear of the right hip was followed by its isolated revision

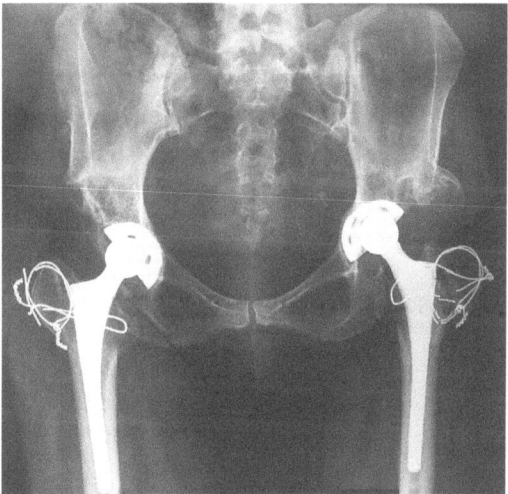

Fig. 9.63   The last follow-up radiograph when the patient was 56 years. The prostheses were stable, 20 years after primary implantation and 9 years after the exchange of the right polyethylene

9.11   Case 13

This female patient was born in 1952 with CHD of the left hip. At the age of 8 years, she was operated in a paediatric centre. There is no information for the type of operation. She was limping since then. We first examined her at the age of 28 years, when she started to have hip pain, which was gradually increasing. THR was postponed until the patient reached the age of 41 years. Preoperatively, a 3D CT scan was needed to definitely classify, this borderline case between low and high dislocation, in B2 subtype of low dislocation. A hybrid Opti-Fix type THR was performed, in 1993. Twenty-three years after surgery, she remains without hip pain or limping and she has a normal life (Figs. 9.64–9.70).

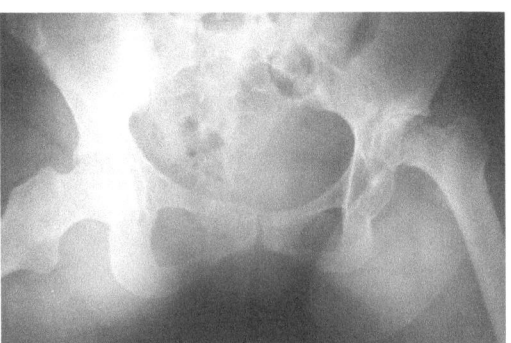

Fig. 9.64 Radiograph at the age of 28 years

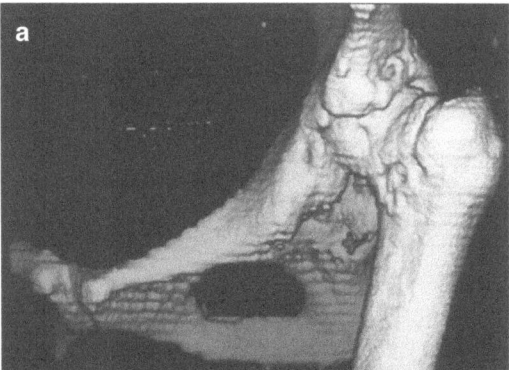

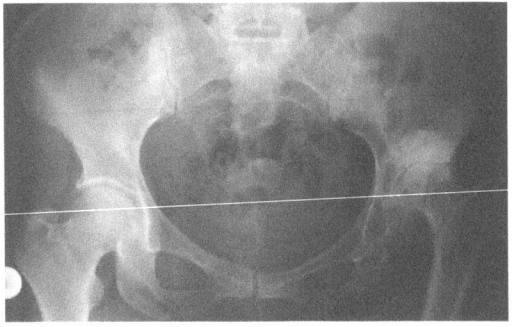

Fig. 9.65 Preoperative radiograph when the patient was 41 years old presenting a borderline hip between low and high dislocation

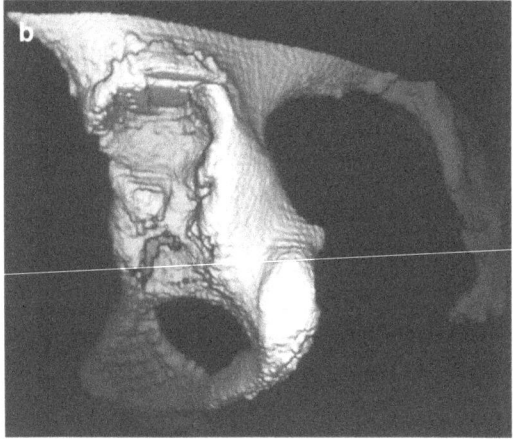

Fig. 9.66 3D CT scan confirmed the diagnosis of B2 subtype low dislocation of the left hip (**a**) with and (**b**) without the femoral head

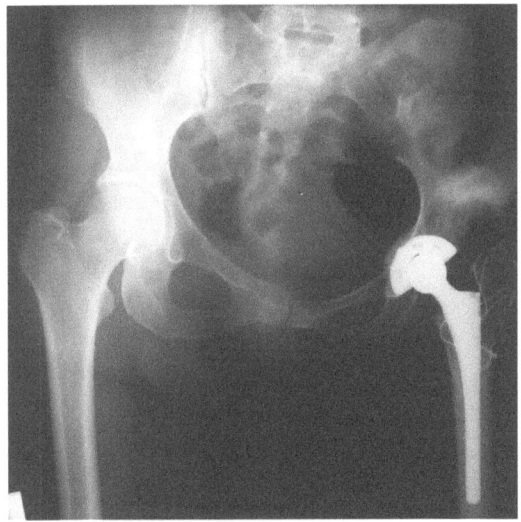

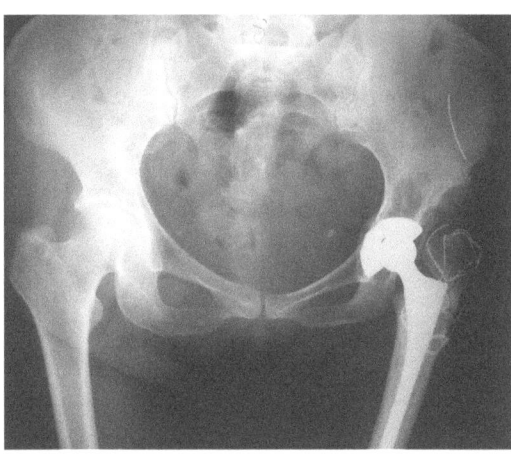

Fig. 9.69 One year later, a broken wire had migrated proximally and was considered as needing no treatment

Fig. 9.67 Early postoperative radiograph

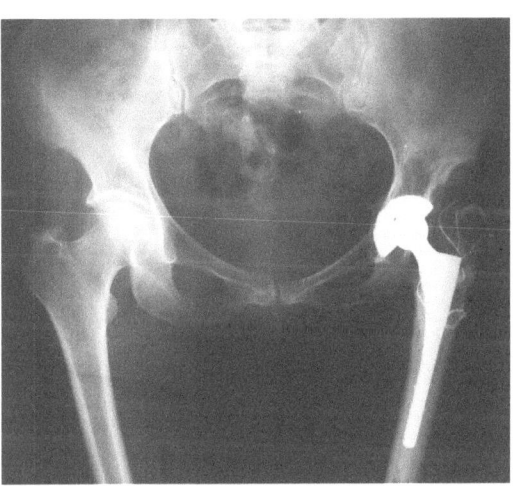

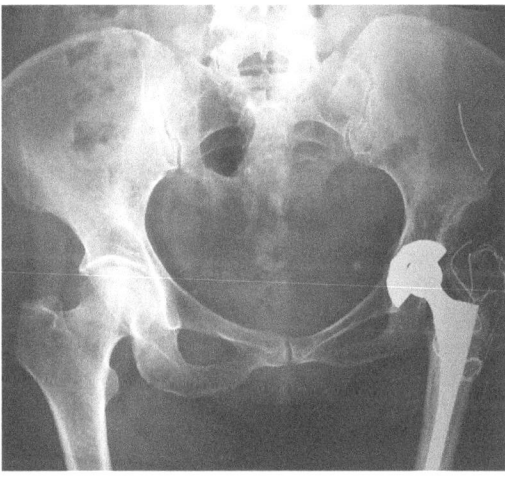

Fig. 9.70 The latest follow-up radiograph, 23 years post-operatively with THR in place. The broken wire is at the same place without any ill effect

Fig. 9.68 Seventeen years after THR

Appendix: Key Messages and Lessons Learned

Key Messages and Lessons Learned

- THR is an exceptionally significant procedure. It should be performed by experienced surgeons, in well-organised orthopaedic centres, only when it is absolutely indicated: "Not too early, not too late".
- The term "total hip replacement" (THR) is more accurate than "total hip arthroplasty" (THA) because it reminds that this is an irreversible procedure in which the destroyed joint is removed and replaced by an artificial one.
- Patients' lifetime follow-up is mandatory to advise them for their lifestyle and to early detect the need for revision, before extended bone stock loss makes revision more complicated.
- While the decision for primary THR is taken in consultation with the patient, the decision for the time of revision is surgeon's responsibility: "Not too early, not too late".
- The assessment of the outcome of a THR and the selection of the appropriate time for revision requires even more experienced surgeons.
- Radiographic evidence of loosening, even migration of the acetabular component, is likely to be asymptomatic, while the same alterations in the femoral component are more likely to be symptomatic.
- The availability in the market of spare parts of a THR is a moral and legal obligation of the orthopaedic industry. This requirement is not always respected and often compels the surgeon to pursue other more complicated solutions, which may be against the patient's health and public economics.
- THR is one of the most successful and cost-effective orthopaedic procedures. Even the pioneer methods of THR have overpassed 40 years of survival and can be used as a benchmark for comparison with the newer methods.
- The choice of the most appropriate method of THR must rely on long-term studies and arthroplasty registries. It should be stressed that studies with short follow-up cannot possibly be used to forecast the long-term outcome of joint replacement.
- Overestimation of secondary parameters concerning THR, such as the minimal invasive surgery techniques, underestimates the importance of this exceptional procedure.
- THR in patients with CHD presents additional technical difficulties, especially in cases with late closed reduction and prolonged immobilisation in plaster in infancy and those with previous osteotomies. For the reconstruction of these hips, wide exposure is needed.
- The transtrochanteric approach, in the previously mentioned cases, not only makes access and reconstruction of the joint easier but may also restores biomechanics, if the distally trochanteric advancement is achieved.
- Charnley insisted that all orthopaedic surgeons should learn the transtrochanteric approach, which may be needed in difficult primary cases and revision operations.
- In high dislocation, shortening of the femur is needed to facilitate hip reduction and to avoid

K. Lampropoulou-Adamidou, G. Hartofilakidis, *Total Hip Replacement*,
DOI 10.1007/978-3-319-53360-5

neurovascular complications. Femoral shortening at the level of the femoral neck is simple and uneventful.

- The reconstruction of the centre of rotation during THR is essential for the restoration of the joint's biomechanics and elongation of the survival of the prostheses.
- Results of THR differ in C1 and C2 subtypes of high dislocation. For that reason, when reporting results of THR in patients with high dislocation, mixing results of the two subtypes may lead to statistical bias.
- THR in patients with concentric idiopathic OA can be postponed for many years, because the deterioration of degenerative changes is slow. On the contrary, eccentric type of idiopathic OA has rapid deterioration, and the patient has to undergo surgery much earlier.
- THR in our patients with inflammatory arthritis was not associated with increased rate of aseptic loosening or dislocation in comparison with THR in patients with OA.
- THR in young patients with advanced stage of AVN of the femoral head is a reasonable option of treatment.
- Even patients who underwent several revisions had the opportunity to enjoy life for a reasonable period of time with functional improvement and without pain.

Relative Publications

1. Hartofilakidis G, Stamos K, Ioannidis TT (1988) Low friction arthroplasty for old untreated congenital dislocation of the hip. J Bone Joint Surg Br 70(2):182–186
2. Karachalios T, Hartofilakidis G, Zacharakis N, Tsekoura M (1993) A 12- to 18-year radiographic follow-up study of Charnley low-friction arthroplasty. The role of the center of rotation. Clin Orthop Relat Res 296:140–147
3. Hartofilakidis G, Stamos K, Karachalios T, Ioannidis TT, Zacharakis N (1996) Congenital hip disease in adults. Classification of acetabular deficiencies and operative treatment with acetabuloplasty combined with total hip arthroplasty. J Bone Joint Surg Am 78(5):683–692
4. Hartofilakidis G, Stamos K, Ioannidis TT (1997) Rotational acetabular osteotomy for severe dysplasia of the hip. J Bone Joint Surg Br 79(3).510

5. Hartofilakidis G, Karachalios T, Zacharakis N (1997) Charnley low friction arthroplasty in young patients with osteoarthritis. A 12- to 24-year clinical and radiographic followup study of 84 cases. Clin Orthop Relat Res 341:51–54
6. Hartofilakidis G (1997) Survival of the Charnley low-friction arthroplasty. A 12-24-year follow-up of 276 cases. Acta Orthop Scand Suppl 275:27–29
7. Hartofilakidis G, Stamos K, Karachalios T (1998) Treatment of high dislocation of the hip in adults with total hip arthroplasty. Operative technique and long-term clinical results. J Bone Joint Surg Am 80(4):510–517
8. Ioannidis TT, Zacharakis N, Magnissalis EA, Eliades G, Hartofilakidis G (1998) Long-term behaviour of the Charnley offset-bore acetabular cup. J Bone Joint Surg Br 80(1):48–53
9. Hartofilakidis G, Karachalios T, Stamos KG (2000) Epidemiology, demographics, and natural history of congenital hip disease in adults. Orthopedics 23(8):823–827
10. Hartofilakidis G, Karachalios T (2000) Total hip replacement in congenital hip disease. Surgical techniques in orthopaedics and traumatology 55-440-E-10. pp 1–7
11. Stamos KG, Karachalios T, Papagelopoulos PJ, Xenakis T, Korres DS, Koroneos E, Hartofilakidis G (2000) Long-term mechanical stability of the impacted morselized graft-cement interface in total joint replacement: an experimental study in dogs. Orthopedics 23(8):809–814
12. Hartofilakidis G, Karachalios T (2003) Idiopathic osteoarthritis of the hip: incidence, classification, and natural history of 272 cases. Orthopedics 26(2):161–166
13. Magnissalis EA, Zinelis S, Karachalios T, Hartofilakidis G (2003) Failure analysis of two Ti-alloy total hip arthroplasty femoral stems fractured in vivo. J Biomed Mater Res B Appl Biomater 66(1):299–305
14. Hartofilakidis G, Karachalios T (2004) Total hip arthroplasty for congenital hip disease. J Bone Joint Surg Am 86-A(2):242–250
15. Hartofilakidis G (2004) Developmental dysplasia of the hip: an unsuitable term. J Bone Joint Surg. Retrieved from website: http://www.ejbjs.org/cgi/eletters
16. Hartofilakidis G, Karachalios T, Karachalios G (2005) The 20-year outcome of the Charnley arthroplasty in younger and older patients. Clin Orthop Relat Res 434:177–182
17. Hartofilakidis G, Yiannakopoulos CK, Babis GC (2008) The morphologic variations of low and high hip dislocation. Clin Orthop Relat Res 466(4):820–824
18. Hartofilakidis G, Georgiades G, Babis GC, Yiannakopoulos CK (2008) Evaluation of two surgical techniques for acetabular reconstruction in total hip replacement for congenital hip disease: results after a minimum ten-year follow-up. J Bone Joint Surg Br 90(6):724–730

19. Vossinakis IC, Georgiades G, Kafidas D, Hartofilakidis G (2008) Unilateral hip osteoarthritis: can we predict the outcome of the other hip? Skelet Radiol 37(10):911–916

20. Yiannakopoulos CK, Chougle A, Eskelinen A, Hodgkinson JP, Hartofilakidis G (2008) Inter- and intra-observer variability of the Crowe and Hartofilakidis classification systems for congenital hip disease in adults. J Bone Joint Surg Br 90(5): 579–583

21. Georgiades G, Babis GC, Hartofilakidis G (2009) Charnley low-friction arthroplasty in young patients with osteoarthritis: outcomes at a minimum of twenty-two years. J Bone Joint Surg Am 91(12):2846–2851

22. Hartofilakidis G, Georgiades G, Babis GC (2009) A comparison of the outcome of cemented all-polyethylene and cementless metal-backed acetabular sockets in primary total hip arthroplasty. J Arthroplast 24(2):217–225

23. Hartofilakidis G, Babis GC (2009) Congenital disease of the hip. Clin Orthop Relat Res 467(2):578–579; discussion 580–571

24. Yiannakopoulos CK, Xenakis T, Karachalios T, Babis GC, Hartofilakidis G (2009) Reliability and validity of the Hartofilakidis classification system of congenital hip disease in adults. Int Orthop 33(2):353–358

25. Karachalios T, Hartofilakidis G (2010) Congenital hip disease in adults: terminology, classification, pre-operative planning and management. J Bone Joint Surg Br 92(7):914–921

26. Georgiades G, Babis GC, Kourlaba G, Hartofilakidis G (2010) Effect of cementless acetabular component orientation, position, and containment in total hip arthroplasty for congenital hip disease. J Arthroplast 25(7):1143–1150

27. Hartofilakidis G, Babis GC, Georgiades G, Kourlaba G (2011) Trochanteric osteotomy in total hip replacement for congenital hip disease. J Bone Joint Surg Br 93(5):601–607

28. Hartofilakidis G, Karachalios T, Georgiades G, Kourlaba G (2011) Total hip arthroplasty in patients with high dislocation: a concise follow-up, at a minimum of fifteen years, of previous reports. J Bone Joint Surg Am 93(17):1614–1618

29. Hartofilakidis G, Babis GC, Lampropoulou-Adamidou K, Vlamis J (2013) Results of total hip arthroplasty differ in subtypes of high dislocation. Clin Orthop Relat Res 471(9):2972–2979

30. Digas G, Georgiades G, Lampropoulou-Adamidou K, Hartofilakidis G (2013) The twenty-year survivorship of two CDH stems with different design features. Eur J Orthop Surg Traumatol 23(8):901–906

31. Karachalios T, Roidis N, Lampropoulou-Adamidou K, Hartofilakidis G (2013) Acetabular reconstruction in patients with low and high dislocation: 20- to 32-year survival of an impaction grafting technique (named cotyloplasty). Bone Joint J 95-B(7):887–892

32. Lampropoulou-Adamidou K, Georgiades G, Vlamis J, Hartofilakidis G (2013) Charnley low-friction arthroplasty in patients 35 years of age or younger. Results at a minimum of 23 years. Bone Joint J 95-B(8):1052–1056

33. Roidis NT, Pollalis AP, Hartofilakidis GC (2013) Total hip arthroplasty in young females with congenital dislocation of the hip, radically improves their long-term quality of life. J Arthroplast 28(7):1206–1211

34. Hartofilakidis G, Babis GC, Lampropoulou-Adamidou K (2014) Congenital hip disease in adults. Springer-Verlag Italia

35. Stathopoulos IP, Lampropoulou-Adamidou KI, Vlamis JA, Georgiades GP, Hartofilakidis GC (2014) One-component revision in total hip arthroplasty: the fate of the retained component. J Arthroplast 29(10):2007–2012

36. Lampropoulou-Adamidou K, Macheras GA, Hartofilakidis G (2015) Bilateral character of total hip replacement does not change the overall survival. Hip Int 25(2):138–141

37. Hartofilakidis GC, Lampropoulou-Adamidou KI, Stathopoulos IP, Vlamis JA (2015) The outcome of 241 Charnley total hip arthroplasties performed by one surgeon 30 to 40 years ago. J Arthroplast 30(10):1767–1771

38. Lampropoulou-Adamidou KI, Tsiridis EE, Kenanidis EI, Hartofilakidis GC (2016) The outcome of 69 recemented hip femoral prostheses performed by one surgeon 22-40 years ago. J Arthroplast 31(10): 2252–2255

39. Karachalios T, Lampropoulou-Adamidou K, Hartofilakidis G (2017) An attempt to throw light on congenital hip disease' terminology and anticipation of clinical outcomes when treated with total hip replacement. Hip Int (accepted)

40. Hartofilakidis G, Lampropoulou-Adamidou K (2016) Lessons learned from the study of congenital hip disease in adults. World J Orthop 7(12):785–792